CLEAN PALEO
real life

EASY MEALS AND TIME-SAVING
TIPS FOR MAKING CLEAN PALEO
SUSTAINABLE FOR LIFE

MONICA STEVENS LE

FAIR WINDS

Inspiring | Educating | Creating | Entertaining

Brimming with creative inspiration, how-to projects, and useful information to enrich your everyday life, Quarto Knows is a favorite destination for those pursuing their interests and passions. Visit our site and dig deeper with our books into your area of interest: Quarto Creates, Quarto Cooks, Quarto Homes, Quarto Lives, Quarto Drives, Quarto Explores, Quarto Gifts, or Quarto Kids.

© 2020 Quarto Publishing Group USA Inc.
Text © 2020 Monica Stevens Le
Photography © 2020 Quarto Publishing Group USA Inc.

First Published in 2020 by Fair Winds Press,
an imprint of The Quarto Group, 100 Cummings Center,
Suite 265-D, Beverly, MA 01915, USA.
T (978) 282-9590 F (978) 283-2742 QuartoKnows.com

Fair Winds Press titles are also available at discount for retail, wholesale, promotional, and bulk purchase. For details, contact the Special Sales Manager by email at specialsales@quarto.com or by mail at The Quarto Group, Attn: Special Sales Manager, 100 Cummings Center, Suite 265-D, Beverly, MA 01915, USA.

24 23 22 21 20   1 2 3 4 5

ISBN: 978-1-59233-951-8
Digital edition published in 2020
eISBN: 978-1-63159-882-1

Library of Congress Cataloging-in-Publication Data

Le, Monica Stevens, author.
Clean paleo real life : easy meals and time-saving tips for making clean paleo sustainable for life / Monica Stevens Le.
ISBN 9781592339518 (trade paperback) | ISBN 9781631598821 (ebook)
1. Cooking (Natural foods) 2. High-protein diet--Recipes. 3. Prehistoric peoples--Nutrition. 4. Cookbooks.
LCC RM237.55 .L43 2020 (print) | LCC RM237.55 (ebook) | DDC 641.5/637--dc23

LCCN 2020000177 (print) | LCCN 2020000178 (ebook)

Design: Kelley Galbreath
Cover Image: Monica Stevens Le
Page Layout: Galbreath Design
Photography: Monica Stevens Le and by Madeline Broderick, Sarah Zimmerman, and Rikki Fore on pages 6, 10, 186, and 188.

Printed in China

The information in this book is for educational purposes only. It is not intended to replace the advice of a physician or medical practitioner. Please see your health-care provider before beginning any new health program.

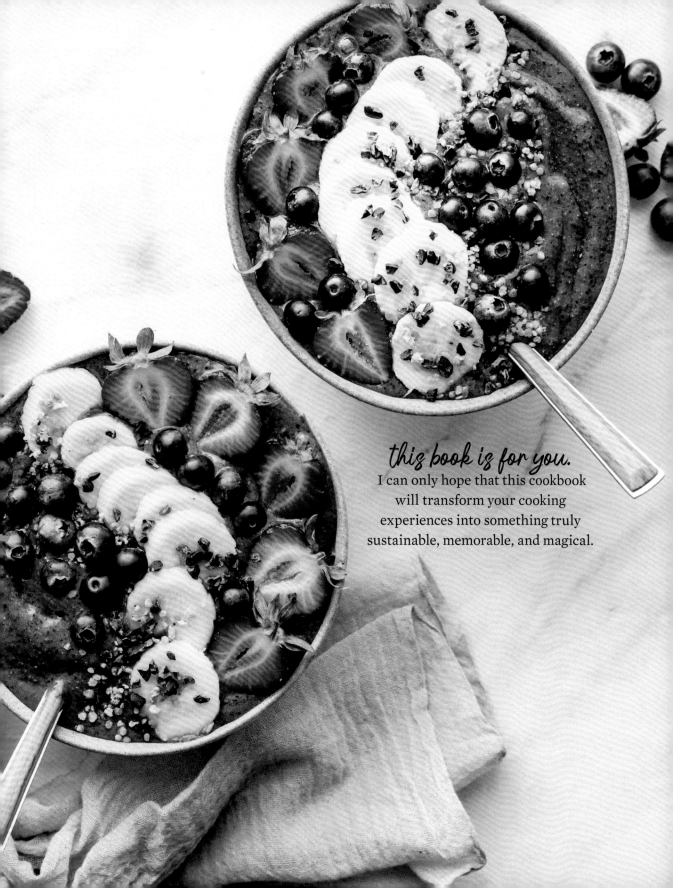

this book is for you.
I can only hope that this cookbook
will transform your cooking
experiences into something truly
sustainable, memorable, and magical.

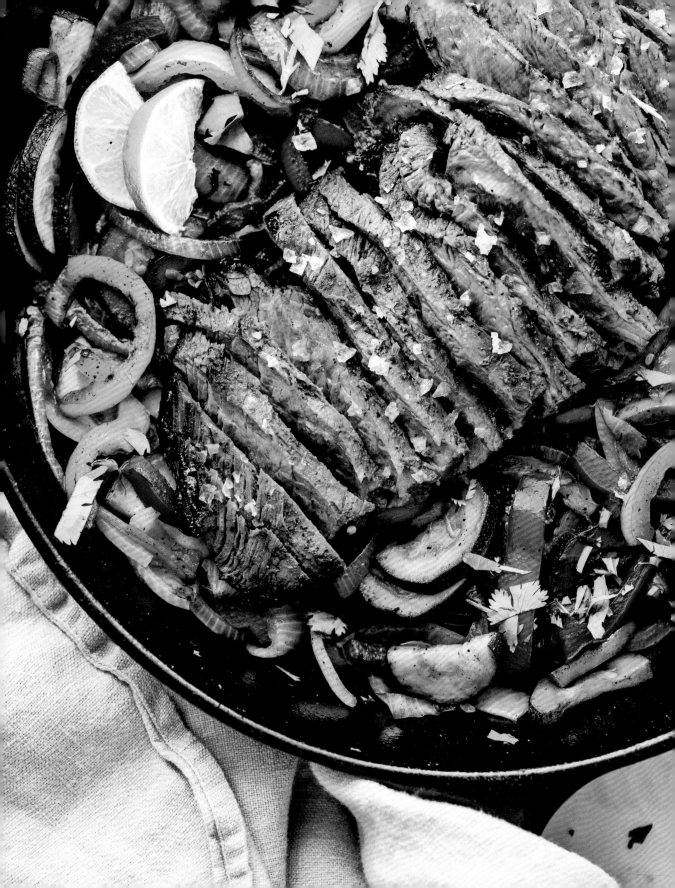

contents

Introduction: My Story | 7

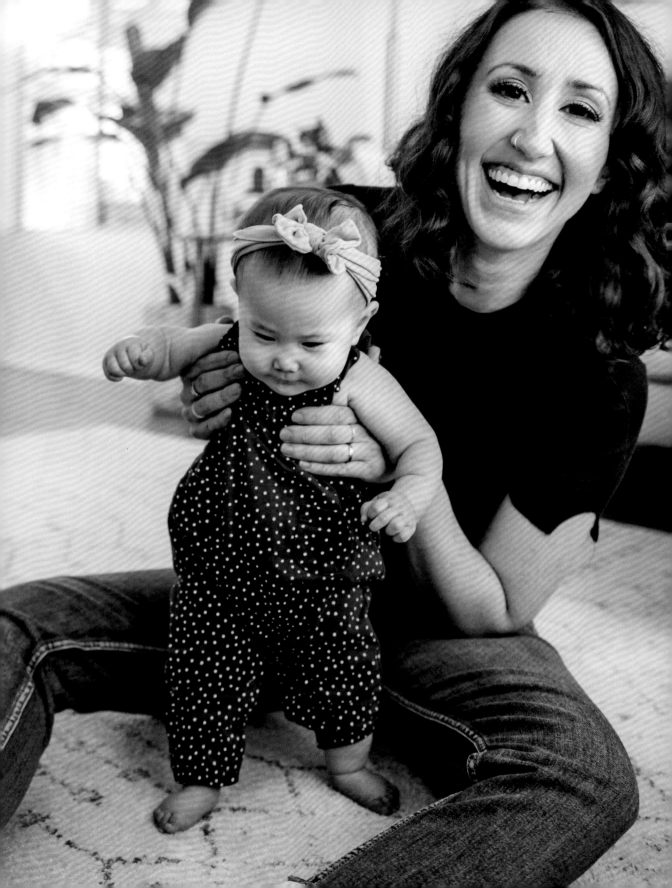

my story

HI, HELLO, HEY! I'M SO HAPPY TO HAVE YOU HERE WITH ME. It makes my heart sing that you have purchased my book and want to improve your health, wellness, and spirit by creating delicious meals in your kitchen. It takes tremendous courage and strength to take charge of your lifestyle in this way, and I absolutely cannot wait to hear from you after trying out my recipes.

First and foremost, I can't talk about eating Clean Paleo without getting into the reasons behind why I started eating this way in the first place. Let's go back to 2011. That was a really big year for me. It was the year I left my job at a big-chain coffee shop, and with it, a whole lot of foods that didn't serve me well. Nothing I ate made me feel great, and I didn't realize that I had accepted feeling pretty crappy all the time as my "normal" and everyday reality.

You see, when you've felt the same way every day for years on end, you forget that it's not how you *should* feel. I remember thinking to myself: "Should I have this little energy after a full night's rest?" or "I can't even zip up my pants after eating a burrito . . . but I'm sure everyone experiences this." I felt that maybe it was just something I would "get over" as time went by. Luckily, I didn't have to endure this insecure and shallow self-acceptance for too long because I stumbled across Clean Paleo eating later that year.

I began eating Clean Paleo in order to figure out which foods truly made me feel like my best self. I'm not only talking about physically feeling and performing at my best. I'm speaking to the emotional state of mind I am in after sitting down and having a meal. Let me explain.

INTUITIVE EATING

About a year into eating this way, I came to the realization that I wanted to eat more foods—and eat them more intuitively. What I mean by this is that once I knew which foods made me feel great and which did not, I didn't have to be so restrictive about my diet. Instead, I could make intentional choices about what I put in my body. With the knowledge I'd acquired through eating Clean Paleo for so long, I understood that I didn't need to deprive myself consistently in order to feel good about myself and the food choices I was making. Because I *knew* how a certain food would make me feel, I could choose to eat it without any surrounding guilt.

A goal of eating intuitively—using Clean Paleo as a template—is to be able to connect to food in a more harmonious and supportive way. As human beings, we are not meant to compartmentalize the very thing that brings us nourishment and life. We simply need to reconnect to our bodies, minds, emotions, and hearts. Once we have gotten to that safe place, we can then find true food freedom and be well on our way to a healthier and more sustainable eating lifestyle.

I live and breathe food. I love cooking and eating; however, I have always tried my best to be very cognizant and mindful about how eating restrictively affects me psychologically. Restrictive eating completely strips the joy from the very thing that brings me so much of it. Making food and sharing it is how I show love to others, and eating restrictively feels like a disservice to not only myself, but also to those around me.

I have found that what works best for me in managing food anxiety is adopting a balanced approach. I use a 30-day Clean Paleo reset whenever I feel like I need to tune up my eating habits and remind myself which foods make my body and mind feel their best. It reminds me of how to eat to thrive. It also reminds me of the opposite—which foods are not enabling me to operate at my full potential. After I'm finished with my 30-day reset, I use the Clean Paleo style of eating as a template to continue creating wholesome, real food dishes in real time. I don't jump back in by eating all the foods that cause me troubles; instead, I reintroduce foods into my diet that I know will make me feel my best. There's no reason to continue eating restrictively (that is, Clean Paleo) unless your body needs to in order to heal from certain ailments, food sensitivities, etc. Thus, you will see a limited number of recipes in the book that do include dairy, grains, or other ingredients that shouldn't be eaten if you are in the strict Clean Paleo elimination phase of your diet. However, if you are not and those foods don't cause issues for you, then there is no reason you can't occasionally incorporate them as part of a whole-foods diet. It's about balance and knowing what works for *your* body. That's what this book is all about.

SHARING CLEAN PALEO FOR A REASON

All of my fondest memories in life stem from experiences around food. I remember at a very young age becoming almost mesmerized by the aromas from my grandmother's kitchen. Who knew that I would turn these vivid childhood memories into a cookbook and career as a successful food blogger?

My main motivation for writing this book was to reach out to anyone who's ever felt as if they couldn't get excited about making and eating food. This is for those who don't feel confident in the kitchen and for those who want to finally enjoy mealtimes. While I knew I wasn't eating the greatest, my journey into Clean Paleo eating didn't stem from a health crisis or an inability to lose weight. Instead, my inspiration to change my lifestyle was driven by the people around me.

Members of my family and several close friends had battled disordered eating for as far back as I can remember. When I say "disordered eating," I mean that these women couldn't enjoy food without feelings of guilt, or they would refuse to try a bite of something if they knew it was high in calories. I have very vivid memories of my mother trying to go down a size or two in jeans when I was growing up. I can easily picture her mentioning "diet" several times a day and turning down certain foods and dishes at family gatherings. I remember thinking, "My mother is so stunning. I know she is perfectly healthy. Why is she doing this to herself?"

Soon after discovering my passion for eating whole, real foods, I wanted to share my findings— and, in turn, joy—with as many people as possible. I wanted to show my friends and family members that eating mindfully and responsibly could truly transform and enrich their lives. I wanted to play a role in helping them break free. That's why I started my blog and why I've created this cookbook.

EATING CLEAN PALEO
IN REAL LIFE

To me, Clean Paleo means creating delicious, mouth-watering recipes that won't make your stomach churn, give you brain fog, cause a blood sugar roller-coaster, or make you feel less than your best after you finish eating them. This means that I've taken some classic recipes and revamped them—sans gluten, grains, dairy, and refined sugar. I've also come up with completely new recipes that are sure to spark your interest and please your taste buds. Wouldn't it be nice to eat a big bowl of cheeseburger soup without the bellyache afterward?

I hope the recipes in this book will inspire you to view cooking as an act of care for yourself and others rather than as a chore. If you have friends or family members who are struggling with health issues and you'd like to help them turn over a new leaf and change their lives, I hope you will serve them a recipe from this book. My wish is that after trying a Clean Paleo version of their favorite dish, they'll realize that giving their diet an overhaul and using real food ingredients doesn't need to be complicated. I created this book in hopes that it would become a valuable resource for people looking to change their relationship with food. I want them to see that they can have gorgeous breakfasts, sumptuous meals, amazing snacks, and yes, even decadent desserts, without feeling deprived.

But my greatest hope in writing *Clean Paleo Real Life* is that you will cook from it so often that you wear this book out. I don't want it to be sitting on your coffee table, collecting dust. This book belongs in your kitchen, covered in sticky notes and sticky fingerprints. I want these recipes to become your new favorites—the dinners you serve to nourish your family or friends at parties and holidays. That is what real life and real cooking means to me.

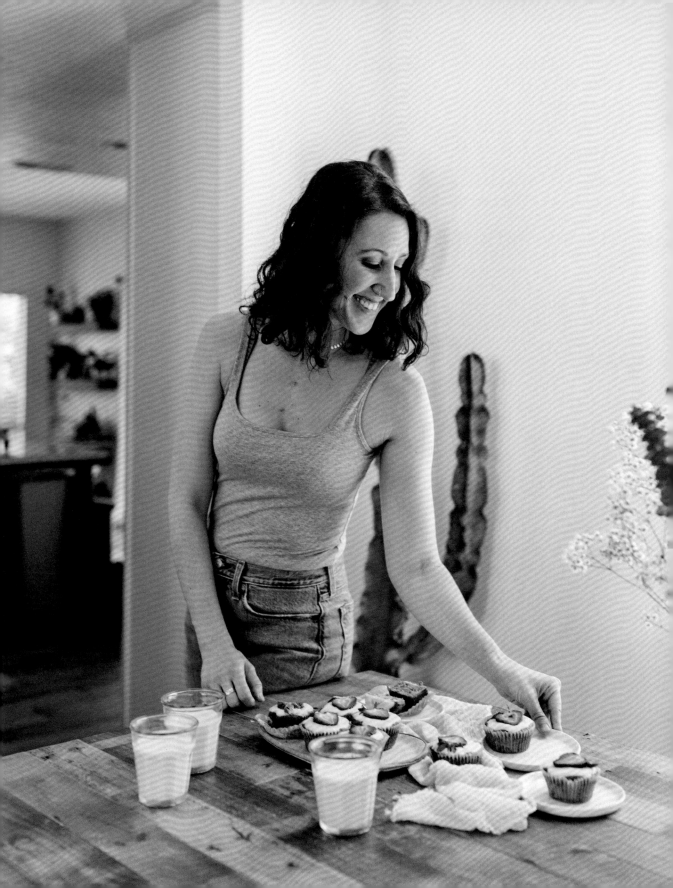

what is the clean paleo lifestyle?

CLEAN PALEO IS MEANT TO BE a 30-day reset to acquaint (or reacquaint) your body and mind with the foods that work best for you. But we're not meant to eat this restrictively forever. This is real life we're talking about, and it's so much more than diet. This means that in addition to eating whole, clean foods, you need to be very present and mindful of every choice you make during each meal. What do I mean by this?

First, there's no eating over the counter or in front of the television. Mealtime means you sit down and slowly and thoughtfully chew your food. Pay attention to the taste and texture of what you're eating. Turn off screens and other noise distractions that keep you from truly enjoying your meal. Just sit down and give your food the attention it deserves. After all, it is responsible for giving you life and health and well-being. It deserves your undivided attention for the duration of your meal.

Why does eating mindfully matter? When we are truly present and completely in tune with what we are putting into our bodies, we are better able to distinguish between hunger and satiety cues. We're not being distracted by anything that could throw off our ability to discern these cues with certainty and confidence. When we can accurately recognize that we are full, we can better recognize when we are truly hungry—and avoid turning to food for reasons other than physical sustenance.

Many of us seek comfort from food for many reasons. It is common practice to eat when we are bored, frustrated, emotionally exhausted, or generally stressed out. Chronic stress can increase the production of our hunger hormones and cravings for typical comfort foods that are high in fat and/or sugar. This is why it is so beneficial to tune into what our minds and bodies are telling us about our relationship with food.

So, what can you eat? Here's a list of real foods, including many options for each category. But keep in mind that you're not limited to *only* these foods during your reset (and beyond).

- **FRUIT:** apples, pears, avocados, berries (strawberries, blueberries, blackberries, raspberries), apricots, grapefruit, cherries, kiwi, lemons, limes, oranges, papaya, peaches, plums, pineapple, pomegranates, tangerines, tomatoes, melons, mangoes, olives, plantains, dates, figs, bananas, grapes, grapefruit, oranges, nectarines

- **VEGETABLES:** winter and summer squash (acorn, butternut, spaghetti, Delicata, pumpkin, zucchini), kale, spinach, collard greens, mustard greens, Swiss chard, asparagus, beets, peppers (bell, jalapeño, shishito), bok choy, broccoli, Brussels sprouts, cabbage, carrots, cauliflower, cucumber, eggplant, garlic, green beans, jicama, lettuce (butter, red, romaine, frisée, arugula, green leaf), mushrooms, onions, parsnips, sugar snap peas and snow peas, sweet potatoes and yams, turnips, radishes, daikon, rutabaga, shallots, artichokes, okra, sprouts, endive, leeks

- **MEATS:** grass-fed beef (ground, steaks), bacon (check labels for added sugar and nitrates), pastured pork (ground, chops, sausage), organic chicken and turkey (ground, sausage, whole, breasts and thighs), deli meat (check labels for additives)

- **SEAFOOD:** wild-caught fish, scallops, shrimp, mussels, clams, crab, etc.

- **EGGS:** cage-free and organic, if possible

- **NUTS AND SEEDS:** almonds, Brazil nuts, cashews, macadamia nuts, pine nuts, pecans, pistachios, walnuts, pumpkin seeds, sesame seeds, hemp seeds, flax seeds, chia seeds

- **COOKING FATS AND OILS:** grass-fed clarified butter (ghee), coconut oil, extra virgin olive oil, avocado oil, sesame oil, lard, palm oil, tallow, duck fat

- **BEVERAGES:** water, tea, coffee, coconut water, mineral water, seltzer water

What should you avoid? During your reset, you'll want to stay away from these items—remember, it's only 30 days! Once you reset, you can start reintroducing them, one group at a time.

- **ADDED SUGAR IN ALL FORMS:** honey, maple syrup, agave nectar, molasses, corn syrup, raw or refined sugar (white, brown, coconut, etc.), Xylitol, Erythritol, monk fruit, Stevia, date syrup, sugar alcohols (ingredients typically ending in -ol), etc. Carefully read labels, as sugar is added to a wide variety of products.

- **ALCOHOL:** this includes cooking with spirits, wine, and beer.

- **GRAINS:** all pasta products, cereals, wheat, rice, quinoa, millet, buckwheat, oats, corn, amaranth, and rye. Read your labels diligently. You will see ingredients like wheat germ, rice flour, corn, etc. in many things. Avoid them all.

- **LEGUMES OF ANY KIND:** all beans, peanuts, shelled peas, chickpeas, and lentils. Stay away from soybeans and soy-based products like soy sauce, miso, tofu, tempeh, and edamame. Look out for soy lecithin on food labels.

- **DAIRY IN ANY FORM:** cow's, sheep's, and goat's milk dairy products, including cream, cheese, yogurt, kefir, ice cream, sour cream, creamer, frozen yogurt, etc.

- **MSG, SULFITES, CARRAGEENAN, AND ANY- THING YOU CAN'T PRONOUNCE:** Check labels for additives like these, as they won't make you feel great and you should avoid them.

WHAT HAPPENS AFTER 30 DAYS? REAL LIFE.

This book is meant to be your resource for Clean Paleo recipes to use during your reset, as well as tried and true favorites that you can look to for reintroducing some of those foods you couldn't eat during your reset.

There are going to be days and occasions when you want to treat yourself. Embrace those feelings. There is no such thing as "cheating" on your way of eating. This isn't a monogamous partnership. Rather, your relationship with food will evolve as your health, life cycles, and many other factors shift. What you are trying to do is achieve a sustainable food-centric lifestyle after your reset. This is where Clean Paleo meets Real Life. How can we even talk about sustaining a lifestyle and way of eating if you're constantly talking about having "cheat" days?

By *choosing* to avoid using words with negative connotations—like "cheating"—we allow ourselves to occasionally indulge, which is a healthy and balanced approach to food. However, indulgence can sometimes come with negative self-talk and feelings of guilt, inadequacy, and failure. All I can say about that is this: It will take many months (sometimes even years) of practice in order to achieve ultimate food freedom.

For example, consider a scenario you might relate to: After your reset, you reach for a box of your favorite chocolate chip cookies while having a girls' night with your besties, and you polish off the entire thing. One of your friends then says, "Wow, I hope this is your cheat day. Are you going to the gym tomorrow to work those off?" Instead of allowing these comments to break you down and trigger feelings of guilt, worry, and sadness, try reframing it this way instead: Yes, you ate a whole box of cookies. But you also just finished 30 days of eating exclusively whole foods and you did so thoughtfully and intentionally. Eating a box of cookies in the moment isn't going to completely derail all the progress you made during your 30 days.

Push past whatever negative feelings your friend's comments might have triggered for you. Simply respond, "I don't believe that I was cheating on anyone or anything. I may or may not go work out tomorrow, but I don't need to work anything 'off.' I really enjoyed all those cookies, and I probably won't feel the need to indulge again for a while. Thanks for your concern, though!" By acknowledging your friend's commentary, you're letting her know that you heard her, and have processed what she has said, but you are also not letting it make you feel ashamed or like a failure for eating.

HOW TO HANDLE REINTRODUCTIONS

After your 30-day reset, you can start reintroducing some foods to see how they make you feel. My recommendation would be to add one reintroduced food at a time and pay attention to how it makes you feel over the course of one day. To make it easier for you, I created nearly half the recipes in this cookbook with the intention of reintroducing a particular "off limits" food back into your diet. Most recipes will highlight just one reintroductory food item at a time so you can really pay attention to how the food you've just eliminated for 30 days makes you feel. I recommend waiting about a week between reintroducing new foods.

For example, it would be challenging to understand how dairy makes you feel if you've just reintroduced it into your diet by eating a bowl of peanut butter chocolate chip ice cream. If your stomach is bothering you afterward and you have acne flare-ups, you'll wonder if it was the sugar or the dairy. Maybe it was the peanut butter. You won't know because you reintroduced several foods at once. That's why I'm using the one-at-a-time strategy throughout this cookbook. However, there are a handful of recipes that have more than one reintroductory food, and I recommend trying out these recipes after each of the featured food groups have been successfully reintroduced. Look for labels at the top of each of recipe so you know at a glance what type of reintroduced food is included in the recipe.

SET YOURSELF UP FOR SUCCESS

Whether you're just starting your journey into eating Clean Paleo, or you've just completed your 30-day reset, prepare to do the following. It will help make your reset and your transition out of the reset smoother.

Stock Up

What should you keep stocked in your pantry? Here is a list of items I always have on hand when I am doing a Clean Paleo reset, but they're also great to have at the ready for any time. Having a well-stocked pantry makes it easier to cook a meal on any given day without feeling as if you have to run to the store all the time. Many of these ingredients are used in the recipes in this book. As always, be sure to read all labels to look for sugar, noncompliant oils, and/or other additives.

- ☐ Capers and olives
- ☐ Broth (vegetable, chicken, beef)
- ☐ Fish sauce
- ☐ Coconut aminos
- ☐ Canned coconut milk and coconut cream
- ☐ Dill pickles
- ☐ Marinara sauce
- ☐ Salsa (pico de gallo, salsa verde, etc.)
- ☐ Dijon mustard
- ☐ Sun-dried tomatoes
- ☐ Ginger paste
- ☐ Tomato paste
- ☐ Fire-roasted peppers
- ☐ Minced garlic
- ☐ Harissa
- ☐ Canned tomatoes
- ☐ Canned fish (tuna, salmon, sardines, oysters)
- ☐ Vinegar (white, balsamic, rice, red wine, apple cider)
- ☐ Nut and seed butters (almond butter, cashew butter, sunflower seed butter)
- ☐ Alternative flours (almond, coconut, tapioca, arrowroot)
- ☐ Approved cooking fats and oils
- ☐ Collagen peptides

Educate Yourself (and Plan Accordingly)

During your Clean Paleo reset, do not recuse yourself from social outings and gatherings. Instead, if you're planning a dinner date or heading out to a new restaurant with coworkers or friends, look up the menu online and figure out what's going to work for you. Even better, call the restaurant if you have any questions or concerns about certain items. (It also gives the restaurant staff a heads-up that you have dietary needs.) Walking into that restaurant with a plan will make executing that plan stress free.

Get Friends and Family on Board

There's nothing better than having the support of friends and/or family while eating Clean Paleo. This is especially true if it is your first go-around. If you've been invited for a night out with close friends who may poke fun at (or not entirely grasp) your new lifestyle, ask them if you can invite your sister along, who just so happens to be eating this way with you! Having that support system right by your side when you're tempted to make unwise food decisions will prove to be tremendously helpful.

Or, how about hosting a Clean Paleo dinner party at your home? It's a great way to show the people you love what you've been up to. After seeing how many delicious things they *can* eat during this informative reset, your guests won't focus as much on the foods to be avoided. And they may even be tempted to join you for your next round!

Seek Out New, Healthy Food You Love

If you've ever perused a menu and dismissed a rather delicious-sounding salad because you didn't know what a main ingredient was, or you feel as if your food options at home are limited because you don't know what a lot of vegetables taste like, it's time to take a trip to the farmers' market! What's so wonderful about the farmers' market is that you can generally ask to try a sample of anything a vendor is selling.

After you've hit the market a few times, your dining-in and dining-out experiences will be a lot more fun and a lot less limiting. Make it a goal to find a few recipes that include items you've never seen before. After trying something new for the first time, you'll feel less intimidated by other recipes that include that same item. And you'll expand the number of foods you have to choose from, which is both exciting and freeing.

Eat Seasonally

This goes hand in hand with checking out local farmers' markets. One of the best parts about eating seasonally is that you can save a lot of money. When you seek out produce that's at its peak growing season and availability, it is going to cost less. What's more, when food is grown closer to you, it doesn't spend a ton of time traveling to make its way to a market near you. This means less energy consumption, which contributes to poor air quality. And I absolutely love anything low-maintenance I can do to reduce my carbon footprint.

Another perk? When food is in season, it tastes the best and is at its healthiest. Foods that are harvested out of season are generally picked before they reach peak flavor because time needs to be allotted for travel. Think of a hard grocery store tomato in May that costs four dollars versus a juicy farm-stand tomato in August at a fraction of the cost; those hard tomatoes are picked before their vitamin C (and flavor) has had a chance to fully develop. The result is food that is more expensive because of the amount of time/labor, distance, and the number of people who have been involved in the process.

Shop Smart

Do your grocery shopping twice a week. This ensures that you'll be planning meals at least two or three days ahead of time, while keeping the possibility of food spoilage very slim. While you're at the grocery store, do your best to stick to the perimeter of the store, where the real food (produce, meat and seafood, eggs, nuts and seeds, etc.) are typically found. At major grocery stores, the middle aisles are where you are going to find the processed food items.

When you head to the market, bring a shopping list and a copy of the recipes you'd like to make for the next few days. Bust out that dusty highlighter and highlight what you need. Better yet, download an app on your phone that allows you to create personalized lists. Read through the recipes and check off what you already have at home and what you'll need to purchase.

Befriend Prep Work

Wash, dry, and cut any produce needed for meal prep over the next few days after you finish grocery shopping and store it in the refrigerator. Otherwise, the amount of prep work required for some dishes (along with the cook time) can seem like a tall order, especially after a long day at work, and you might become tempted to reach for something less healthy that's easier to make. Prepping a day or two ahead will save you a lot of time and plenty of sanity.

Store Food in Portions

I'm not talking about limiting yourself to restrictive, "diet-size" portions of food. Rather, by portioning out meals in to-go containers when you're finished cooking, it will make grabbing breakfast, taking lunch to go, and heating up dinner a whole lot easier!

YOUR NEW COMMUNITY AWAITS!

The best part of eating Clean Paleo is the undeniable amount of support you will have within the Paleo community. Social media is a great place to find like-minded individuals who are following a Clean Paleo lifestyle as well. You'll find such unity, unwavering support, and encouragement among those who are on a Clean Paleo eating journey alongside you. You can share anecdotes, struggles—and now, recipe success stories!—with others who just might need encouragement. Now let's get cooking!

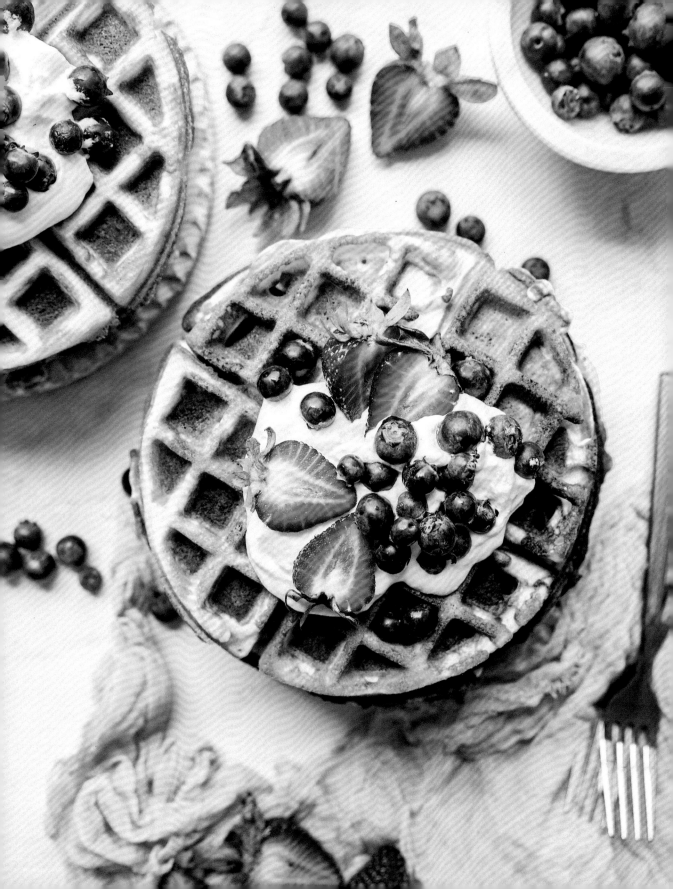

CHAPTER 2

breakfast & snacks

HERE'S MY THOUGHT ON BREAKFAST: *completely necessary*. I understand that not all of us are wired the same way, but I can't even begin to function if I haven't filled up my belly in the morning. I think that people get burnt out on breakfast because they're always thinking of the same old breakfast food. Take eggs, for example. I love me some eggs, and I'm not saying you won't find egg-based dishes in this chapter—but you're going to find so much more! There are awesome breakfast dishes that are fit for a cutesy Sunday brunch and others that are best for on-the-go, fast-paced weekday mornings. You can't go wrong, and I've included a lot of variety for those who can't face the same thing every day. Cashew Cheese Chilaquiles, Paleo/Keto Waffles, and Beef & Bacon Breakfast Bowls are some of my favorites.

You're also going to find many snack items in this chapter, but they're so hearty you might as well eat them for breakfast. Sink your teeth into Paleo Açai Bowls and Rice Flour Banana Muffins—seriously, they both are so delicious, you're going to be excited about snacks (and breakfast!) again.

◀ Paleo/Keto Waffles, page 32

PREP TIME:
5 minutes

COOK TIME:
10 minutes

YIELD:
2 servings

cauliflower rice n'oatmeal

3 cups (540 g) cauliflower rice

1 cup (240 ml) full-fat canned coconut milk

¼ cup (60 ml) unsweetened almond or cashew milk

¼ cup (40 g) hemp seeds/hearts

2 tablespoons (30 ml) pure maple syrup

2 teaspoons (4.6 g) ground cinnamon

1½ teaspoons (7.5 ml) pure vanilla extract

Pinch of pink or kosher salt

2 scoops collagen peptides or 1 serving protein powder

This cauliflower n'oatmeal is chock-full of so many nutrient-dense foods, you won't miss your regular bowl of morning oats. Enjoy it first thing in the morning, after an intense workout, or as a snack. Be sure to sprinkle on your favorite toppings like mixed toasted nuts, fresh or dried fruit, coconut flakes, or coconut whipped cream.

1 Add the cauliflower rice, coconut milk, and almond or cashew milk to a medium saucepan and stir together over medium-high heat.

2 Add the hemp, syrup, cinnamon, vanilla, and salt. Simmer until thick and quite creamy, about 10 minutes, stirring every few minutes.

3 Once thickened, stir in the collagen peptides or protein powder.

4 Remove from the heat. Use an immersion blender to blend it a few times.

5 Divide between two bowls and top with your favorite fixings.

PREP TIME:
5 minutes

COOK TIME:
25 minutes

YIELD:
10 muffins

SWEETENER / GRAIN

rice flour banana muffins

½ cup (120 ml) unsweetened nondairy milk

⅓ cup (80 ml) unsweetened applesauce

¼ cup (60 ml) grass-fed butter or coconut oil, melted and cooled

¼ cup (60 ml) pure maple syrup

1 teaspoon (5 ml) pure vanilla extract

1 cup (120 g) brown rice flour

½ cup (60 g) blanched almond flour

1½ teaspoons (7 g) baking powder

¼ teaspoon kosher salt

1½ bananas, chopped (keep them separate)

2½ tablespoons (27 g) chia seeds

These muffins are light, fluffy, and super delicious. Everyone in the family will love them, just as my daughter loves to nom on one or two as a snack. They taste great plain at room temperature or toasted with a little slather of butter or ghee, if that's your jam. They also freeze well, so be sure to double up on the batch if you want some for grab-and-go!

1   Preheat the oven to 375°F (190°C) and adjust the oven rack to the middle position. Line a cupcake or small muffin tin with 10 parchment liners and very lightly spray with extra oil.

2   In a large mixing bowl, whisk together the milk, applesauce, butter or coconut oil, syrup, and vanilla until well combined.

3   Sift in the rice flour, almond flour, baking powder, and salt. Stir lightly until everything has been well incorporated, but do not overmix!

4   Fold in 1 chopped banana and the chia seeds.

5   Fill each parchment liner about three-quarters full. The batter should divide evenly among the 10 liners. Top off with the remaining half banana.

6   Bake until a toothpick inserted into the center comes out clean, or 22 to 25 minutes. Let them cool in the pan for 10 minutes and then transfer to a wire rack to cool completely.

PREP TIME:
15 minutes +
marinating time

COOK TIME:
45 minutes

YIELD:
4 servings

GRAIN / DAIRY

cashew cheese chilaquiles

CHICKEN
3 tablespoons (45 ml)
    avocado oil
4 cloves garlic, minced
1 tablespoon (15 ml)
    fresh lime juice
1 tablespoon (7.5 g)
    chili powder
1 teaspoon (2.5 g)
    ground cumin
1 teaspoon (2.5 g) paprika
1 teaspoon (6 g) kosher salt
¾ teaspoon dried oregano
¼ teaspoon black pepper
1 pound (450 g) boneless,
    skinless chicken thighs

CHILAQUILES
¼ cup plus 2 tablespoons
    (60 ml plus 30 ml)
    avocado oil, divided
8 corn tortillas, cut into
    quarters
1 teaspoon (6 g) kosher salt
1 cup (240 ml) 15-Minute
    Blender Salsa (page 179)
4 large eggs
½ cup (45 g) Cashew
    Cheese (page 174)
¼ cup (40 g) finely diced
    red onion
2 avocados, diced
½ cup (45 g) finely chopped
    Cotija cheese (optional)
Handful fresh cilantro,
    finely chopped

Chilaquiles are a fabulous breakfast dish that includes fried corn tortilla pieces, cooked in salsa, and then topped off with cheese. You can easily make chilaquiles at home that will make you quickly forget about any chilaquiles you have ever ordered at a restaurant. For starters, the cashew cheese is so creamy and delightful, you're going to want it as a dip for anything and everything. It pairs well with the spicy, tangy chicken, and all the flavors combined are a serious symphony of deliciousness. This would be a fabulous meal to make for brunch or breakfast on a slow morning—plan ahead and marinate the chicken before you head to bed.

1 To make the chicken, in a medium bowl, whisk together the oil, garlic, lime juice, chili powder, cumin, paprika, salt, oregano, and pepper. Transfer to a shallow glass container or resealable plastic bag and add the chicken, making sure it's submerged in the mixture. Cover or seal and refrigerate for at least 2 hours or overnight.

2 When you are ready to work with the chicken, preheat the oven to 425°F (220°C) and adjust the oven rack to the middle position. Line a rimmed baking sheet with aluminum foil or parchment paper.

3 Transfer the chicken to the prepared baking sheet. Pour the extra marinade over the chicken. Roast until it is cooked through to 165°F (74°C), about 30 minutes. Remove from the oven to let cool before slicing into strips or cubes.

4 Meanwhile, to make the chilaquiles, in a large skillet over medium-high heat, heat ¼ cup (60 ml) of the oil until tiny bubbles start to form, 2 to 3 minutes. Add the tortillas, taking care not to overcrowd them. Fry until crisp throughout, about 3 minutes, and transfer to a paper towel–lined plate. Sprinkle with the salt. Set aside the chips and discard the oil.

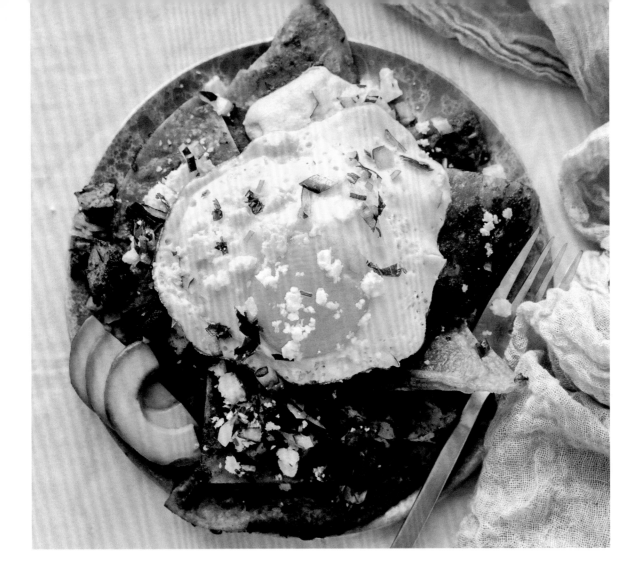

5 Add 1 tablespoon (15 ml) oil to the skillet, and add the salsa. Cook over medium heat until quite warm, about 2 minutes, and then add the crispy tortilla quarters. Make sure the tortillas are fully coated in salsa on both sides and cook until the tortillas soften a bit, 3 to 5 minutes; they should not break down at all.

6 Meanwhile, prepare the eggs. Heat another medium skillet over medium heat for 2 minutes and add the remaining 1 tablespoon (15 ml) oil. Add the eggs and cook until the yolks have set, 3 to 4 minutes. Set aside.

7 Evenly divide the chips and salsa among serving plates. Top the tortillas with the chicken, dividing evenly among plates. Top off with the cashew cheese, fried eggs, onion, avocado, cheese (if using), and cilantro.

PREP TIME:
25 minutes
COOK TIME:
35 minutes
YIELD:
4 servings

ultimate breakfast sheet pan

2 tablespoons (30 ml) avocado oil, divided

3 cups (10 ounces or 280 g) Brussels sprouts, trimmed and halved

3 carrots, sliced

1 large zucchini, thinly sliced

1 small yellow onion, sliced

5 ounces (140 g) cremini or baby bella mushrooms, coarsely chopped

Kosher salt, to taste

Black pepper, to taste

6 strips bacon, cut into large chunks

6 cloves garlic, minced

4 large eggs

1 avocado, diced

Chopped fresh parsley (or favorite herb), for garnish

I simply adore how low-maintenance it is to create a one-pan breakfast dish. This is especially true when that breakfast includes bacon, eggs, and all kinds of vegetables that will leave you feeling satisfied (and excited that you ate so many veggies for breakfast!). Get a jump start on it by cutting all the veggies before you go to bed. This breakfast is topped off with diced avocado and fresh herbs, and it's the absolute perfect way to start your morning.

1 Preheat the oven to 425°F (220°C) and adjust the oven rack to the middle position.

2 Pour 1 tablespoon (15 ml) of the oil onto a rimmed baking sheet and spread it around evenly using a pastry brush or paper towel.

3 Arrange the Brussels sprouts, carrots, zucchini, onion, and mushrooms on the baking sheet, but do not overcrowd (use a second sheet pan, if necessary). Drizzle with the remaining 1 tablespoon (15 ml) oil and sprinkle sparingly with salt and pepper (the bacon will add quite a bit of saltiness).

4 Arrange the bacon over the veggies. Roast for 15 minutes. Remove from the oven and sprinkle the entire pan with the garlic. Give everything a good stir and return the pan to the oven until the veggies are cooked through and the bacon looks crisp, another 15 minutes.

5 Create four wells for the eggs in the veggies. Carefully crack an egg into a small bowl and pour into a well. (This will ensure you do not break the egg.) Repeat for all the eggs. Return the pan to the oven and bake until the eggs have cooked to your desired level of doneness. (I remove mine after 6 minutes.)

6 Remove from the oven and serve immediately, topped with the avocado and parsley.

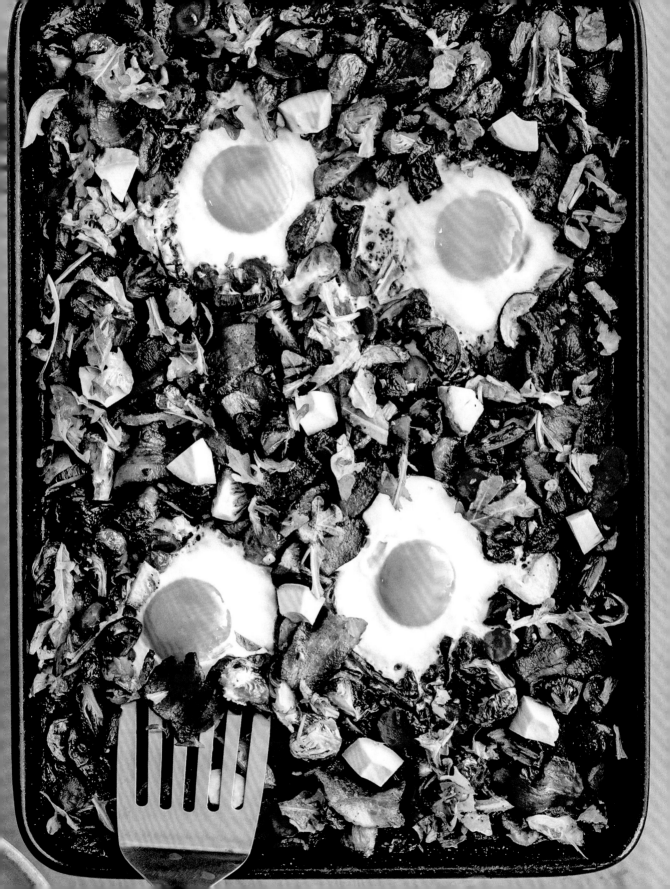

PREP TIME:
15 minutes

COOK TIME:
40 minutes

YIELD:
4 to 5 servings

beef & bacon breakfast bowls

POTATOES AND ASSEMBLY

1½ pounds (675 g) Yukon gold potatoes, cut into 1-inch (2.5 cm) cubes

2 tablespoons (30 ml) avocado oil

Kosher salt, to taste

Black pepper, to taste

3 cups (113 g) lightly packed arugula

1½ tablespoons (22 ml) extra virgin olive oil

1 avocado, sliced, for garnish

Chopped fresh parsley, for garnish

PATTIES

1½ pounds (675 g) 90/10 ground beef (see Notes)

4 strips bacon, cooked and diced

2 tablespoons (8 g) chopped fresh parsley

1½ teaspoons (9 g) kosher salt

1 teaspoon (6 g) black pepper

1 teaspoon (5 g) garlic powder

1 teaspoon (3.6 g) crushed red pepper flakes

½ teaspoon smoked paprika

¼ teaspoon dried thyme

2 tablespoons (30 ml) ghee or avocado oil, divided

RANCH

½ cup (120 ml) Clean Paleo Mayo (page 176)

How great would it be on those hectic mornings to have breakfast prepped that required only a few minutes to reheat and assemble? Sounds like a win to me. These filling breakfast bowls are loaded with healthy fats and delicious greens. The peppery arugula pairs so well with the creamy ranch dressing, savory beef and bacon patties, and crispy potatoes—and they get a double bonus for not having eggs. Yum!

1 Preheat the oven to 425°F (220°C) and adjust the oven rack to the middle position. Line a baking sheet with parchment paper.

2 To make the potatoes, in a large bowl, toss the potatoes with the avocado oil, using your hands or a spoon, until they are evenly coated. Spread in an even layer onto the baking sheet. Sprinkle with salt and pepper.

3 Roast until they begin to turn golden brown, 25 to 30 minutes. Turn the oven to a low broil for 4 minutes, turning the baking sheet 180 degrees halfway through.

4 Meanwhile, to make the patties, in a large bowl, combine the beef, bacon, parsley, salt, black pepper, garlic powder, red pepper, paprika, and thyme. Mix well with your hands, and make sure everything has been evenly dispersed. Form into 8 to 10 patties, ½ to ¾ inch (13 to 19 mm) thick.

5 Heat a large skillet over medium to medium-high heat and add 1 tablespoon (15 ml) of the ghee or oil. Once the skillet has heated up for 2 minutes, add half the patties and fry until cooked through and browned on the outside, 2 to 3 minutes on each side. Keep a close eye on them. Transfer the patties to a plate and cook the rest of the patties with the remaining 1 tablespoon (15 ml) oil, repeating the same steps.

6 Meanwhile, make the ranch dressing. In a small bowl, whisk together the mayo, coconut milk, dill, garlic powder, and a pinch of salt and pepper. Set aside.

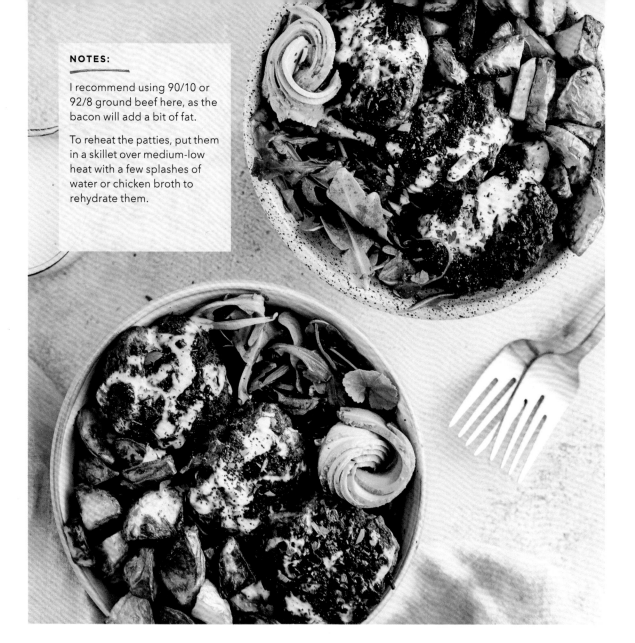

NOTES:

I recommend using 90/10 or 92/8 ground beef here, as the bacon will add a bit of fat.

To reheat the patties, put them in a skillet over medium-low heat with a few splashes of water or chicken broth to rehydrate them.

½ cup (120 ml) full-fat canned coconut milk
1 teaspoon (1.3 g) fresh dill, finely chopped
½ teaspoon garlic powder
Kosher salt, to taste
Black pepper, to taste

7 In another large bowl, toss together the arugula with the olive oil and a pinch of salt and pepper. Use your hands to massage the oil into the leaves and set aside.

8 To serve, divide the crispy potatoes and arugula among plates and set 2 patties on each. Drizzle with the ranch dressing, and top with the avocado and parsley.

PREP TIME:
5 minutes + chill time

COOK TIME:
1 minute

YIELD:
8 bars

SWEETENER

½ cup (75 g) raw cashews

½ cup (75 g) walnuts

½ cup (75 g) pumpkin seeds

⅓ cup (50 g) unsweetened raisins

5 tablespoons (30 g) collagen peptides

3 tablespoons (33 g) chia seeds

3 tablespoons (36 g) flaxseeds

2 tablespoons (15 g) cacao nibs

½ cup (120 g) creamy cashew butter

3 tablespoons (45 ml) coconut oil

2 tablespoons (30 ml) pure maple syrup

1 teaspoon (5 ml) pure vanilla extract

NOTE:

Get creative with the nuts and seeds. Feel free to use almonds, pecans, sunflower seeds, etc.

high-protein paleo granola bars

What if I told you that in 10 minutes you could make home-made paleo granola bars that are as nutritious as they are delicious? This awesome mixture of nuts and seeds tastes fabulous with cacao nibs, creamy cashew butter, and raisins. Feel free to get creative and swap out some of the nuts or seeds for your favorites. These bars are perfect with breakfast, as a snack, or to grab and go, go, go!

1 Line an 8 x 8-inch (20.5 x 20.5 cm) baking dish with parchment paper.

2 In the bowl of a food processor, add the cashews, walnuts, pumpkin seeds, raisins, collagen, chia, flax, and cacao nibs. Pulse several times until coarse throughout. Transfer the mixture to a large bowl and set aside.

3 In a small saucepan, combine the cashew butter, coconut oil, syrup, and vanilla over low heat. Mix thoroughly until smooth and creamy throughout, about 1 minute.

4 Add the wet ingredients to the dry and give everything a good stir.

5 Transfer the mixture to the prepared baking dish. Press down with the bottom of a glass, jar, or your fingertips to pack it into the bottom of the dish, creating an even base. If it's too sticky, lightly wet your fingertips.

6 Place in the refrigerator to set overnight. Cut into 8 bars with a sharp knife. Store in an airtight container in the refrigerator for up to 10 days.

PREP TIME:
15 minutes

COOK TIME:
15 minutes

YIELD:
12 muffins

breakfast frittata muffins

12 large eggs
¾ cup (180 ml) nondairy milk
¼ cup (37 g) flaxseed meal
1 teaspoon (3 g) garlic powder
¾ teaspoon kosher salt (see Notes)
2 large handfuls arugula
1 cup (150 g) green beans, steamed and cut into 1-inch (2.5 cm) pieces

Wouldn't it be wonderful to have a quick and easy go-to breakfast for both you and your kids? These muffins will be loved by the whole family. They are full of greens and flaxseed meal for extra fiber that everyone needs. They are creamy, quick to make, and absolutely de-lish! Perfect for toddlers *and* adults!

1 Preheat the oven to 350°F (180°C) and adjust the oven rack to the middle position. Line a muffin tin with parchment liners and lightly spray with oil.

2 In a large bowl, whisk together the eggs, milk, flaxseed meal, garlic powder, and salt, if using. Fold in the arugula and green beans.

3 Divide the mixture among the muffin tins, filling each about three-quarters full.

4 Bake until the eggs have puffed up and look cooked, 14 to 18 minutes. A slight jiggle in the center is okay. Place the tin on a wire rack to cool.

5 Store muffins in an airtight container in the refrigerator for up to 1 week. Reheat in a toaster oven.

NOTES:

These muffins do not freeze or thaw out well.

If you're making these for a baby, omit the salt.

PREP TIME:
15 minutes +
overnight

COOK TIME:
35 minutes

YIELD:
about 4 cups
(950 g) oatmeal;
about 2½ cups
(595 g) jam

———

SWEETENER / GRAIN

JAM
2 pounds (900 g) fresh
   strawberries, hulled
¼ cup (60 ml) pure maple
   syrup
2 tablespoons (28 g) chia
   seeds
1½ tablespoons (22 ml)
   fresh lemon juice

OATS
2¼ cups (595 ml) nondairy
   milk
½ cup (120 g) cashew butter,
   plus more for serving,
   if desired
¼ cup (40 g) chia seeds
3 tablespoons (45 ml) pure
   maple syrup
1½ teaspoons (7.5 ml) pure
   vanilla extract
2 cups (180 g) old-fashioned
   oats (see Notes)

NOTES:

———

Check labels to ensure
your oats are processed
at a gluten-free facility.

This recipe will also
work with quick and
steel-cut oats.

overnight cashew butter oats with homemade jam

I would argue that there could be nothing better than waking up in the morning and realizing breakfast has already been taken care of. This recipe comes pretty close to that. I absolutely love how low-maintenance it is, and you're going to flip over the strawberry jam. I love to top these oats off with some extra cashew butter, diced fruit, coconut flakes, or chopped nuts. You can't go wrong, and I don't doubt you'll be licking your bowl clean, either.

1 To make the jam, in a medium saucepan, combine the strawberries and syrup over medium heat. Cover and carefully bring to a simmer, stirring every minute or so. After about 5 minutes, the strawberries will begin to release their juices. Use a potato masher to smash them down.

2 Add the chia and lemon juice and reduce the heat to medium-low. Continue cooking, uncovered, stirring every few minutes or so. After about 30 minutes, the mixture will have thickened quite a bit. Remove it from the heat now, as it will continue thickening as it cools.

3 Let the jam cool for 10 to 15 minutes before transferring to another vessel or jar. This will make a lot of jam, so you will have plenty left over to store in the refrigerator for up to 2 weeks.

4 To make the oats, in a large glass bowl or plastic container, combine the milk, cashew butter, chia, syrup, and vanilla. Stir well with a spoon.

5 Add the oats and give it another good stir. Make sure the oats are completely submerged in the liquid in order to ensure an even setting process.

6 Cover and refrigerate overnight.

7 In the morning, give it another good stir and serve with extra cashew butter (if you'd like) and the homemade jam.

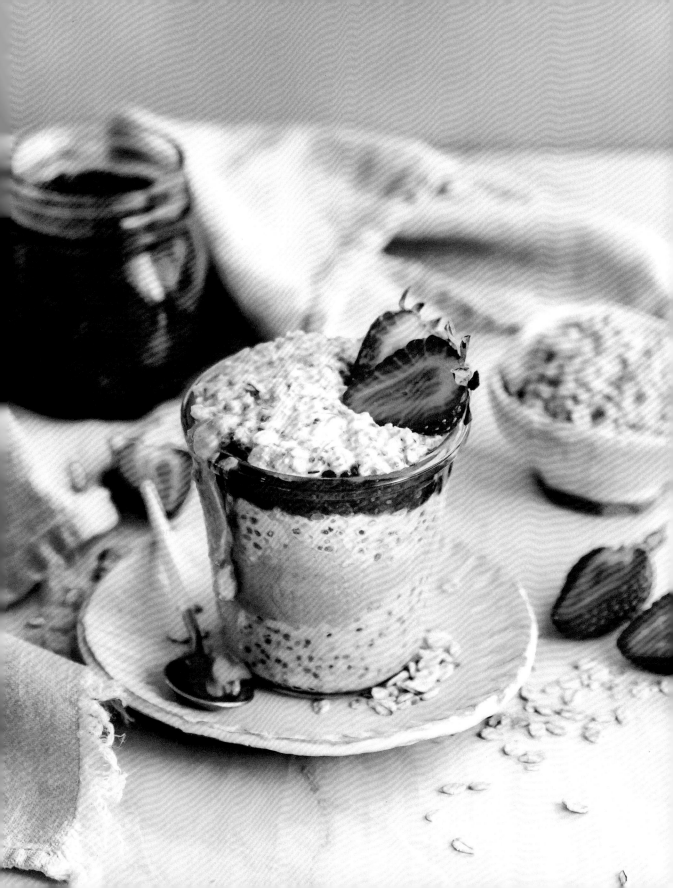

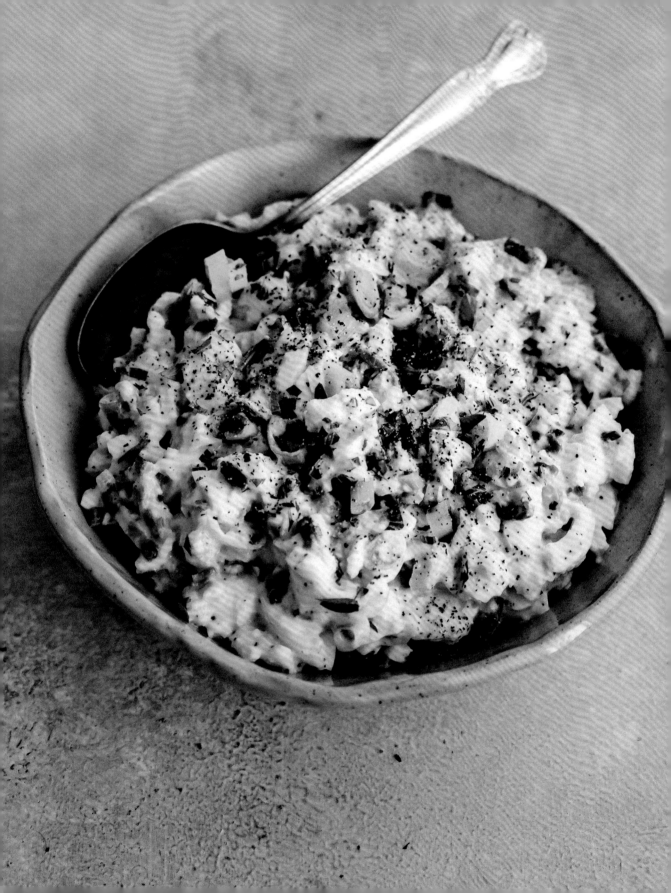

PREP TIME:
15 minutes +
chill time

COOK TIME:
20 minutes

YIELD:
4 servings

soft-boiled egg salad

6 strips bacon
12 large eggs
½ teaspoon kosher salt, plus a pinch, divided
⅔ cup (160 ml) Clean Paleo Mayo (page 176)
⅓ cup (50 g) chopped scallions
1 tablespoon (15 ml) Dijon mustard
¼ teaspoon black pepper
¼ cup (40 g) chopped fresh chives

So what's this recipe doing in the breakfast chapter? Think of it as a bacon and egg mash-up. This Clean Paleo recipe is both easy to make and kid approved. I love having it as a salad with breakfast or lunch, but it's great to have on hand for a quick protein-filled snack. I serve it over a bed of mixed greens or with bell pepper slices or veggie chips. If you aren't on a Clean Paleo reset, feel free to toast up some gluten-free bread and make an awesome egg salad sandwich.

1 Line a baking sheet with parchment paper and add bacon strips in a single layer. Place into a cold oven and set the temperature to 375°F (190°C). Bake until crispy throughout and cooked through to your preference, 22 to 28 minutes. Remove from the oven; once cool, cut into small pieces.

2 Meanwhile, prepare the eggs by placing them in a medium saucepan. Add enough water to cover by 1 inch (2.5 cm). Transfer the eggs back to a bowl and set the saucepan of water over high heat. Once the water is boiling, add a big pinch of salt and very carefully lower in the eggs. Lower the heat to medium-high and cook for 7 minutes. Prepare a big bowl of ice water. Once the eggs are done, transfer them to the ice water bowl and let them cool for 10 minutes.

3 Peel and rinse the eggs in that cold water. Pat them dry. Chop into small pieces and transfer to a large bowl.

4 Add the mayo, bacon, scallions, mustard, remaining ½ teaspoon salt, and pepper. Stir well. Taste for more salt and pepper. Serve immediately, but for best flavor, refrigerate for 2 to 3 hours. Garnish with the chives before serving.

PREP TIME:
5 minutes

COOK TIME:
20 minutes

YIELD:
8 to 10 large waffles

SWEETENER

paleo/keto waffles

1 cup (120 g) coconut flour

1 cup (120 g) tapioca flour

⅓ cup (65 g) granular Erythritol sweetener (see Notes)

1½ teaspoons (7 g) baking powder

1 teaspoon (6 g) kosher salt

4 large eggs, at room temperature

1¼ cups (300 ml) full-fat canned coconut milk

¼ cup (60 ml) ghee or coconut oil, melted

1½ teaspoons (7.5 ml) pure vanilla extract

⅔ to 1⅓ cups (160 ml to 320 ml) water (see Notes)

NOTES:

To make these waffles paleo instead, use ½ cup (100 g) coconut sugar in place of the Erythritol.

You may need less or more water, depending on how fatty and thick your coconut milk is. The batter should be thick but pourable.

I can't wait for you to try these paleo- and keto-friendly waffles. They're incredibly easy to make and take very little time to prepare. Top them with your favorite fixings, like fresh berries, whipped coconut cream, grass-fed butter, maple syrup—or the homemade strawberry jam on page 28. They're also fabulous plain—try them and see for yourself.

1 Preheat your waffle iron according to the manufacturer's directions.

2 In a large bowl, whisk together the coconut flour, tapioca flour, sweetener, baking powder, and salt.

3 In a medium bowl, whisk the eggs. Add the coconut milk, ghee or coconut oil, and vanilla and whisk until well combined.

4 Pour the wet ingredients into the dry and stir them together. At this point, your mixture should be pretty thick, and that's fine! Add in ¼ cup (60 ml) water at a time and keep stirring. Your mixture will be thick like lava, but roll with it for now.

5 Brush or spray a layer of oil onto both the top and bottom of the waffle iron's griddle.

6 Pour enough of the waffle batter into the iron to barely cover the bottom, around ¼ cup (60 ml). You do not want to add too much because your iron will begin to overflow! Cook according to the manufacturer's directions.

7 Depending on the size of your waffle iron, this makes about 8 large waffles. Top with your favorite toppings and serve warm.

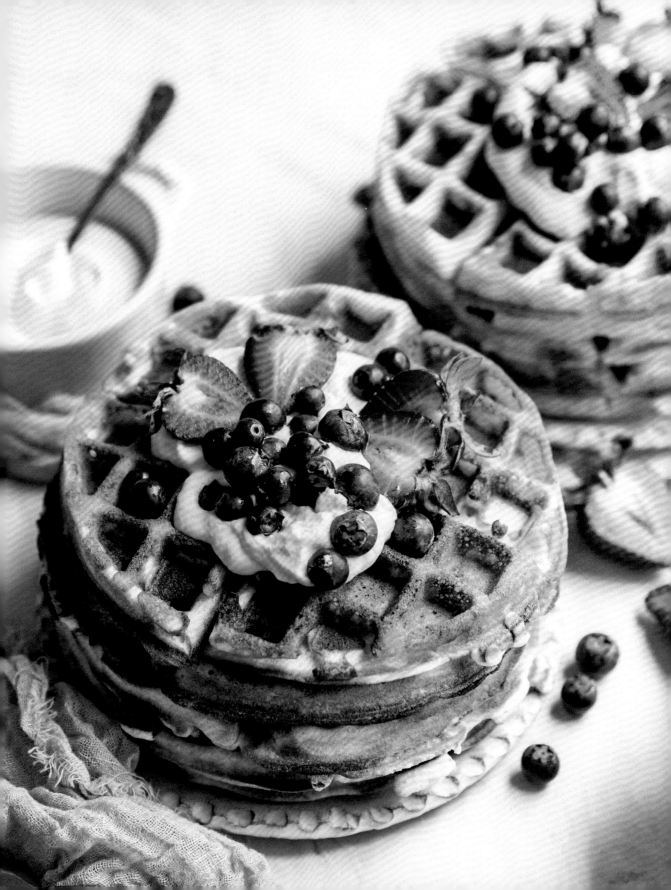

PREP TIME:
5 minutes
COOK TIME:
N/A
YIELD:
2 bowls

paleo açai bowls

1 packet (3.5 ounces [70 g])
 frozen, unsweetened açai
 (see Notes)
1¼ cups (225 g) frozen
 mixed berries
1 small frozen banana
½ cup (120 ml) unsweetened
 coconut or almond milk
 (see Notes)
2 tablespoons (22 g) hemp
 seeds or chia seeds
2 scoops collagen peptides
 (omit for vegan, see Notes)
1 heaping tablespoon
 (15 g) cashew butter
 or almond butter
1 tablespoon (15 ml)
 coconut oil
Toppings of choice (see
 headnote for ideas)

These pretty, fruit-filled bowls are packed with all kinds of
nutrient-dense ingredients, like creamy cashew butter, coconut oil, and hemp seeds. They're the perfect balance of tart
and sweet, and your whole family will love them. I like to
play around with toppings, using strawberries, blueberries,
bananas, cacao nibs, and bee pollen. What a refreshing way
to start the day!

1 In the pitcher of a high-speed blender, add the açai, berries, banana,
 milk, seeds, collagen (if using), nut butter, and coconut oil.

2 Blend on medium-high speed for 1 minute. Scrape the sides or use the
 tamper to make sure everything gets blended well.

3 Pour into two bowls and top with your favorite toppings.

NOTES:

The açai comes already pureed and frozen in individual-serving-
size packages.

This recipe uses coconut milk from a carton, not the canned variety.

If you are omitting the collagen peptides, be sure to make up the thickness
by using an extra ¼ to ⅓ cup (40 to 50 g) frozen berries.

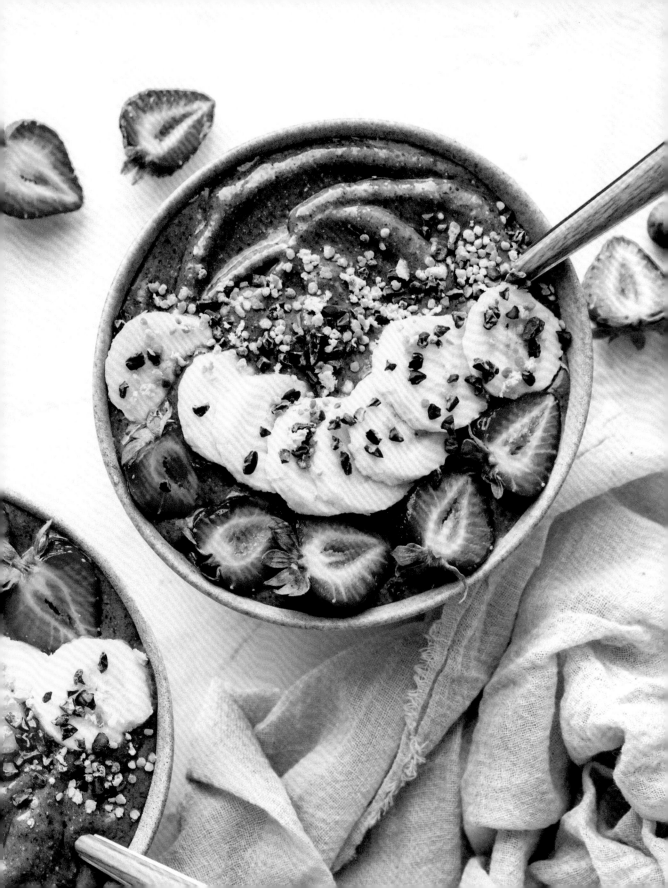

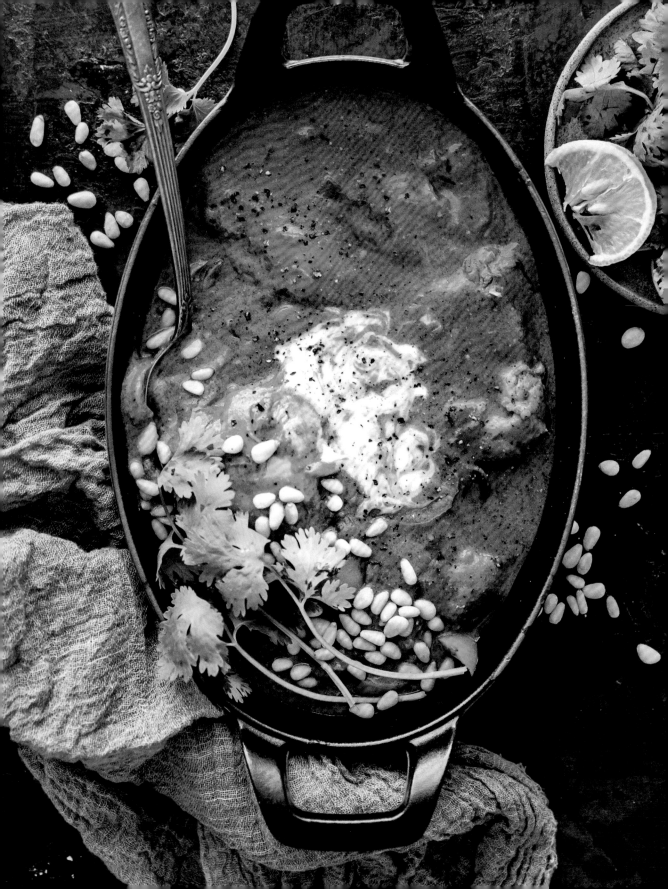

soups & salads

SOUP OR SALAD? IF I'M BEING HONEST, this is a question I don't care to be bothered with. Usually, the options are a bit underwhelming, even at nicer establishments. In this chapter, though, I set out to really change the soup and salad game. I wanted all these recipes to be filling enough to eat on their own as a meal. Here you'll find Greek Salad with Cashew Tzatziki, Salmon Niçoise Salad Wraps, Chicken Korma Stew, and a Low-Carb Cheeseburger Soup.

One of my favorite things about soups and salads is how easy they are to store. If you store the dressing on the side, a salad can keep for several days in the refrigerator. And most soups can be frozen and defrosted, if you want to cook them in batches or if you won't be able to eat the whole recipe in a day or two.

And don't relegate salads to summer and soups to winter. You're going to want to eat these year-round. They are that good. Who says we can only eat soups when it's cold out? I want to feel warm and cozy on pretty much every evening!

◀ Chicken Korma Stew, page 50

PREP TIME:
20 minutes +
marinating time
COOK TIME:
30 minutes
YIELD:
6 to 8 servings

DAIRY

chicken taco salad

CHICKEN
6 tablespoons (90 ml)
  avocado oil
2 tablespoons (30 ml)
  fresh lime juice
1½ tablespoons (22 g)
  chili powder
6 cloves garlic, minced
2 teaspoons (5 g) paprika
2 teaspoons (12 g) kosher
  salt
1½ teaspoons (3.75 g)
  ground cumin
1½ teaspoons (1.5 g)
  dried oregano
½ teaspoon black pepper
2 pounds (900 g) boneless,
  skinless chicken thighs

SALAD
⅔ cup (160 ml) 15-Minute
  Blender Salsa (page 179)
⅔ cup (160 ml) sour cream
  or Greek yogurt
3 romaine hearts, chopped
1 cup (150 g) grape
  tomatoes, halved
¾ cup (65 g) shredded
  Mexican-style cheese or
  favorite cheese blend
Kosher salt, to taste
Black pepper, to taste
2 medium avocados, cubed
⅔ cup (100 g) chopped
  scallions
Handful fresh cilantro,
  chopped

This taco salad is out of this world. The combination of my blender salsa mixed with sour cream makes for the most irresistible dressing. You'll also love the array of flavors and textures of the tangy and spicy chicken thighs, juicy tomatoes, creamy avocado, and cheese. It's like the best deconstructed taco of your life.

1 To make the chicken, in a medium bowl, whisk together the oil, lime juice, chili powder, garlic, paprika, salt, cumin, oregano, and pepper until well combined. Transfer to a shallow glass container or resealable plastic bag and add the chicken, making sure it's submerged in the mixture. Refrigerate for at least 2 hours or overnight.

2 When you are ready to work with the chicken, preheat the oven to 425°F (220°C) and adjust the oven rack to the middle position. Line a rimmed baking sheet with aluminum foil or parchment paper.

3 Transfer the chicken to the prepared baking sheet. Pour the extra marinade over the chicken. Roast until it is cooked through to 165°F (74°C), about 30 minutes. Remove from the oven to cool before slicing into strips or cubes.

4 Meanwhile, to make the salad, in a small bowl, whisk together the salsa and sour cream and set aside.

5 In a large bowl, toss together the romaine, tomatoes, and cheese; alternatively, assemble on a platter. Top with the cooked chicken and drizzle with the salsa sauce. Sprinkle with salt and pepper, to taste. Add the avocados, scallions, and cilantro before serving.

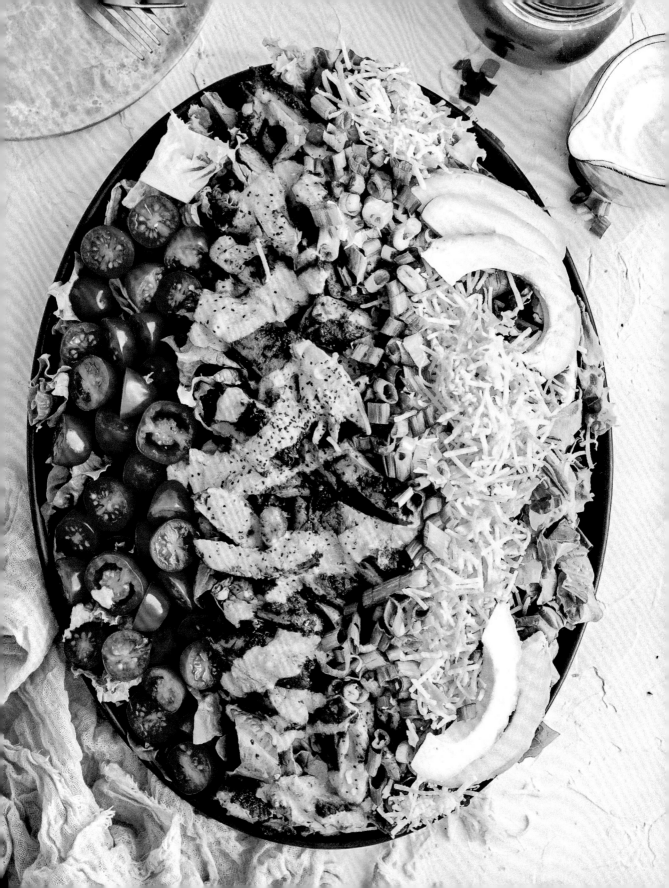

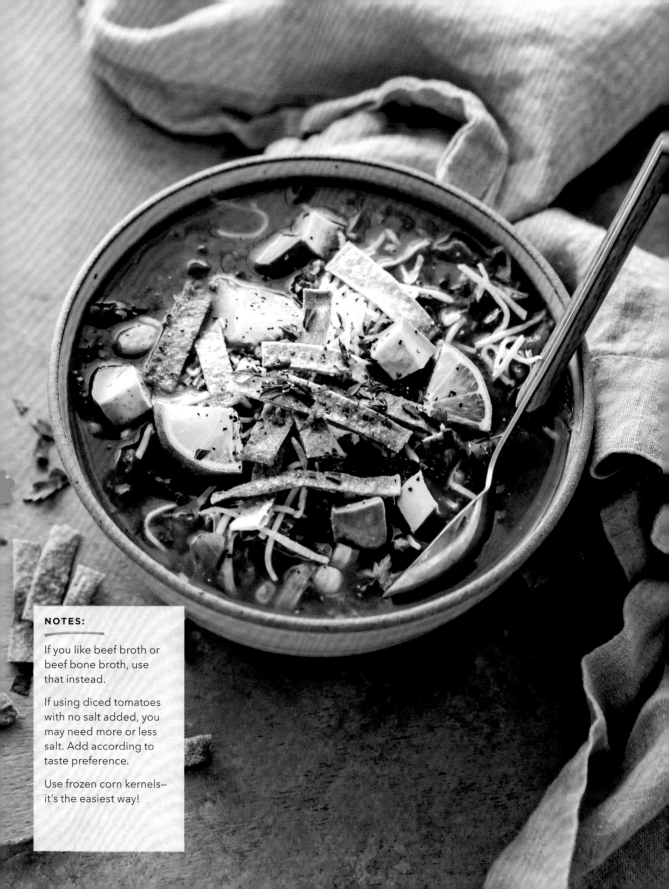

NOTES:

If you like beef broth or beef bone broth, use that instead.

If using diced tomatoes with no salt added, you may need more or less salt. Add according to taste preference.

Use frozen corn kernels— it's the easiest way!

PREP TIME:
15 minutes
COOK TIME:
30 minutes
YIELD:
6 servings

GRAIN

chicken tortilla soup

TORTILLA STRIPS
¼ cup (60 ml) avocado oil
6 small corn tortillas, cut into
¼-inch (6 mm) strips
1 teaspoon (6 g) kosher salt

SOUP
2 tablespoons (30 ml)
avocado oil
1 yellow onion, diced
1 jalapeño, minced (remove
seeds for less heat)
6 cloves garlic, minced
1 quart (1 L) chicken broth
or chicken bone broth
(see Notes)
2 cans (14.5 ounces [435 ml])
diced tomatoes (see Notes)
3 cups (375 g) shredded
cooked chicken
2 cups (250 g) corn kernels
(see Notes)
½ lime, juiced
1 tablespoon (15 g) chili
powder
1 to 2 teaspoons (6 to 12 g)
kosher salt
1½ teaspoons (3.75 g)
ground cumin
1½ teaspoons (7.5 g) smoked
paprika
1 teaspoon (2 g) black
pepper
⅔ cup (160 ml) full-fat canned
coconut milk
Handful fresh cilantro, finely
chopped
Diced avocado, for topping

This warm and comforting soup is going to be your new go-to, especially after you see how simple it is to make. (Save time by using a rotisserie chicken!) The homemade tortilla strips are going to change your life, and I can almost assure you there won't be leftovers (for long, at least). If you already know you have no problem with black beans, you can absolutely throw in a can of those. Oh, and the creamy coconut milk mixed in really takes this soup to the next level, too.

1 To make the tortilla strips, place a large skillet over medium heat and warm the oil for 2 to 3 minutes, or until tiny bubbles start to form. Add the tortilla strips, taking care not to overcrowd them. Fry until crisp throughout, about 3 minutes, and transfer to a paper towel–lined plate. Sprinkle with the salt.

2 To make the soup, place a large Dutch oven or stockpot over medium-high heat and warm the oil for 2 minutes. Add the onion and jalapeño and sauté until they begin to soften, about 5 minutes. Add the garlic and sauté for another minute, stirring frequently.

3 Add the broth, tomatoes, chicken, corn, lime juice, chili powder, 1 teaspoon (5 g) salt, cumin, paprika, and pepper. Bring to a low boil and allow it to boil gently for 5 minutes, stirring occasionally. Add the coconut milk and return to a low boil. Cook for an additional 3 to 5 minutes, stirring occasionally. Add the cilantro and boil for 1 minute more.

4 Taste and add more salt, if needed.

5 Ladle the soup into bowls and top with the tortilla strips, avocado, and more cilantro, if desired.

PREP TIME:
10 minutes +
chill time

COOK TIME:
N/A

YIELD:
6 servings

curried chicken salad in avocado boats

- 2 teaspoons (10 g) curry powder
- ½ teaspoon (2.5 g) kosher salt, plus more to taste
- ½ teaspoon (2.5 g) black pepper, plus more to taste
- ½ teaspoon (2.5 g) dried thyme
- 5 cups (625 g) shredded cooked chicken
- 2 small bell peppers (red, orange, or yellow), finely diced
- 1 small green apple, finely diced
- 1 small red onion, finely diced
- ¾ to 1 cup (180 to 240 ml) Clean Paleo Mayo (page 176)
- 6 avocados, halved, for serving
- ¼ cup (40 g) sliced scallions, for garnish
- 3 tablespoons (12 g) chopped fresh parsley, for garnish

Is there anything better than chicken salad for breakfast, lunch, and dinner? It sounds like overkill, but you won't think so after trying this curried rendition of it made with juicy and succulent chicken thighs, crisp apple, onion, bell pepper, and my Clean Paleo mayo. Feel free to swap the avocado half with a tomato half, or eat the salad with your favorite type of rice, bread, etc.

1 In a large bowl, combine the curry powder, salt, black pepper, and thyme. Add the chicken and use your hands to thoroughly rub the spices into it.

2 Add the bell peppers, apple, and onion and toss until combined.

3 Pour the mayonnaise over the chicken and vegetables and mix thoroughly with your hands, making sure everything is completely coated with the mayo. Taste for additional salt and pepper.

4 Cover the bowl and refrigerate for at least 1 hour before serving.

5 Pile the chicken salad onto the avocado halves. Garnish with the scallions and parsley.

6 Store the chicken salad in an airtight container in the refrigerator for up to 5 days.

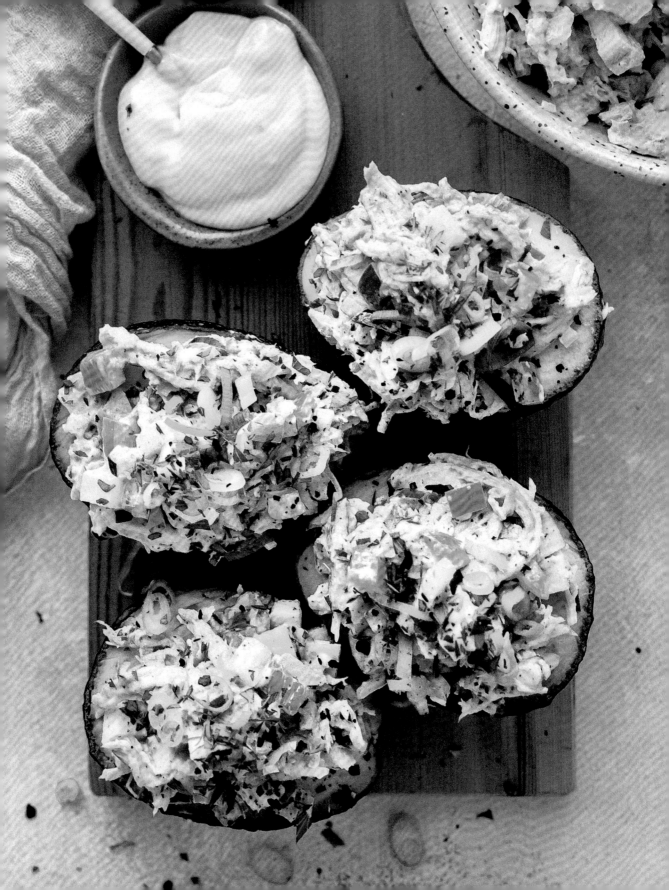

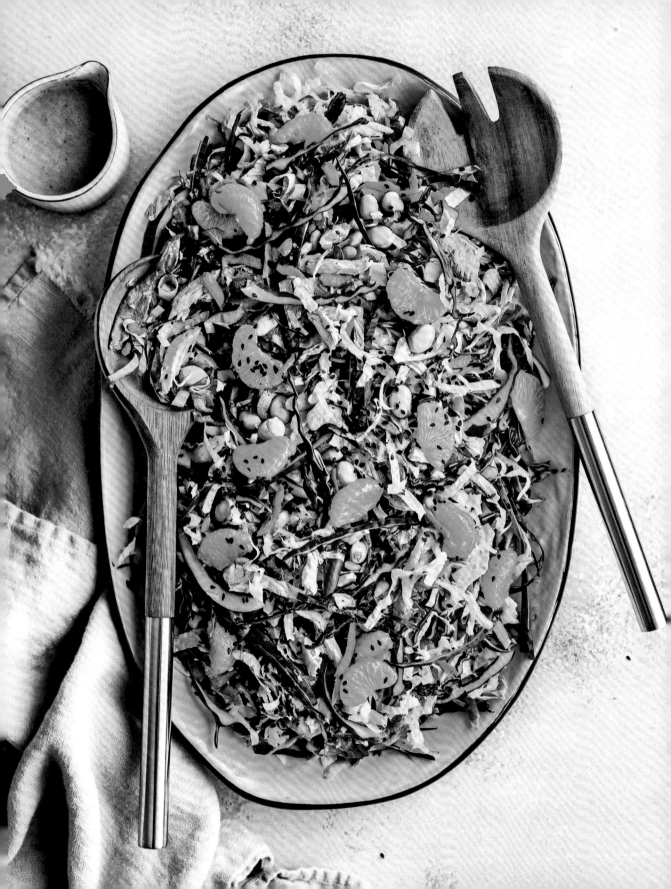

PREP TIME:
20 minutes

COOK TIME:
N/A

YIELD:
6 servings

SOY

chinese chicken salad

DRESSING
¼ cup (60 ml) avocado oil
¼ cup (60 ml) rice vinegar
3 tablespoons (45 ml)
  sesame oil
2 tablespoons (30 ml) Clean
  Paleo Mayo (page 176)
2 tablespoons (30 ml)
  coconut aminos
1 teaspoon (2.7 g) grated
  fresh ginger
1 teaspoon (6 g) kosher salt
½ teaspoon garlic powder
¼ teaspoon black pepper

SALAD
3 cups (375 g) shredded
  rotisserie chicken
3 cups (450 g) thinly
  shredded red cabbage
3 romaine hearts, thinly
  sliced
3 carrots, peeled and grated
1 cup (150 g) shelled
  edamame, steamed
  (omit for Clean Paleo)
1 cup (150 g) canned
  mandarin oranges, drained
1 cup (150 g) raw cashews,
  coarsely chopped
¾ cup (120 g) thinly sliced
  scallions
Black sesame seeds, for
  garnish

Although this fabulous Chinese chicken salad sticks to a some-what traditional ingredient list—edamame, shredded cabbage, mandarin oranges, and cashews—there are no fried noodles. The quick avocado oil dressing gets its kick from fresh ginger and really ties the dish together. You're going to love it.

1 To make the dressing, add the avocado oil, vinegar, sesame oil, mayo, coconut aminos, ginger, salt, garlic powder, and pepper to the pitcher of a blender. Blend until smooth.

2 To make the salad, toss together the chicken, cabbage, romaine, carrots, edamame (if using), oranges, cashews, and scallions in a large bowl.

3 Drizzle the salad with the dressing and toss very well to coat. You may end up using all the dressing, and that's great! Sprinkle with the sesame seeds before serving.

4 If you have leftovers, this salad will not become soggy and inedible after sitting in the refrigerator. Store in an airtight container in the refrigerator for up to 3 days.

PREP TIME:
15 minutes
COOK TIME:
25 minutes
YIELD:
6 servings

the best dang broccoli salad

SALAD
½ pound (230 g) bacon, cooked and crumbled
6 cups (900 g) bite-size broccoli florets
½ medium red onion, thinly sliced
⅔ cup (100 g) sliced almonds
⅔ cup (100 g) unsweetened raisins

DRESSING
¾ cup (180 ml) Clean Paleo Mayo (page 176)
2 tablespoons (30 ml) rice vinegar
1 tablespoon (15 ml) coconut aminos
Black pepper, to taste

There's nothing like a creamy-crunchy broccoli salad, am I right? This is a pretty classic rendition—with bacon, red onion, almonds, and raisins—but the dressing is what really takes it over the moon. Bring it to a potluck, eat it as a side dish, or top it off with your favorite protein for a complete meal. It's fabulous any way you swing it!

1   To make the salad, line a baking sheet with parchment paper and add the bacon strips in a single layer. Place into a cold oven and set the temperature to 375°F (190°C). Bake for 22 to 28 minutes, until crispy throughout and cooked through to your preference. Transfer to a paper towel–lined plate and let cool. Cut or crumble into pieces.

2   To make the dressing, whisk together the mayo, vinegar, coconut aminos, and pepper in a small bowl. Taste for black pepper and set aside.

3   To finish the salad, toss together the bacon, broccoli, onion, almonds, and raisins in a large bowl.

4   Pour the dressing over the salad and toss to thoroughly coat. Taste for seasoning. You may need another tablespoon or two of mayo, depending on your preference for how saturated you'd like the salad.

5   Store for up to 5 days in an airtight container in the refrigerator.

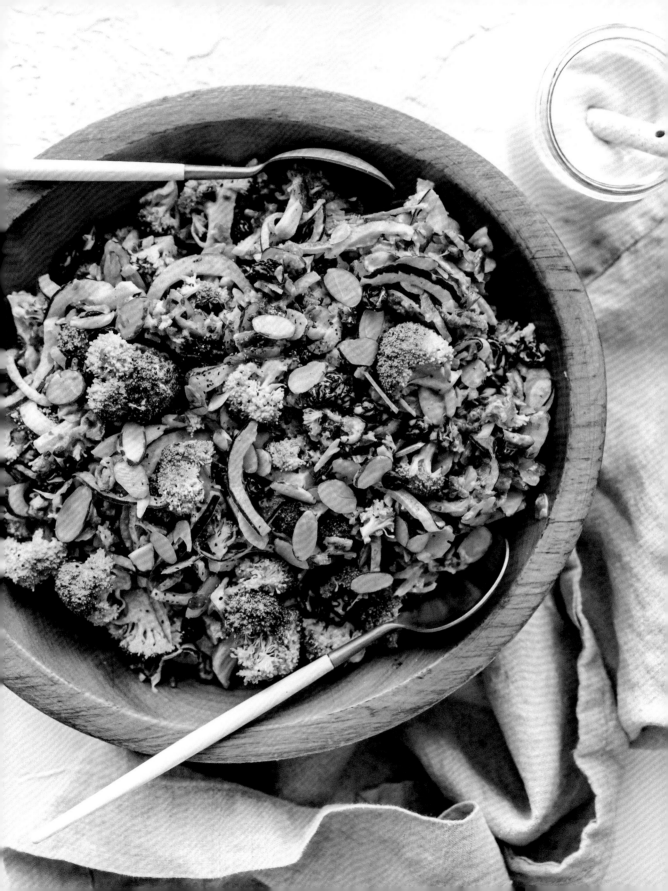

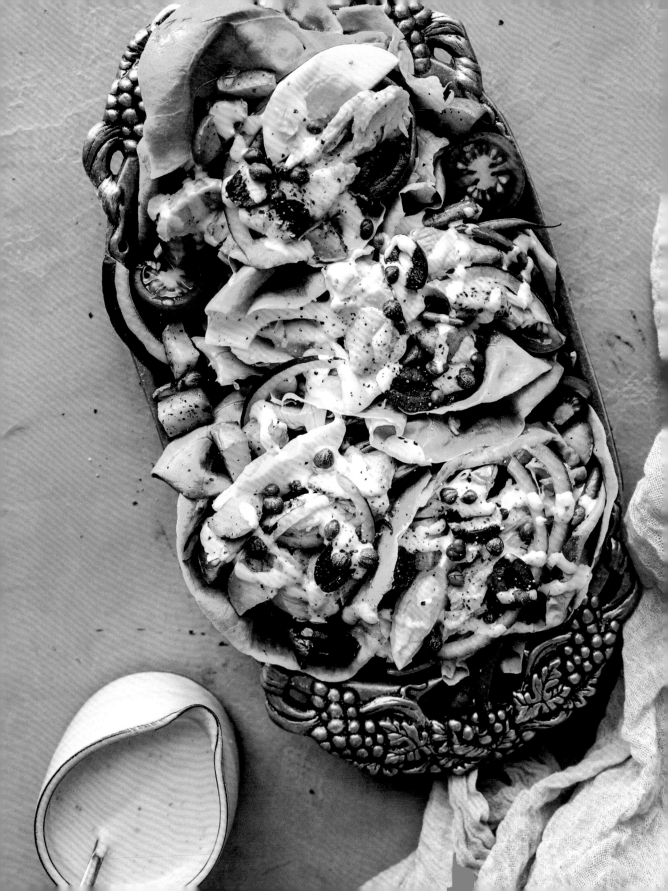

PREP TIME:
20 minutes

COOK TIME:
35 minutes

YIELD:
4 servings

salmon niçoise salad wraps

SALAD

1 pound (450 g) Yukon gold potatoes, cut into 1-inch (2.5 cm) chunks

3 tablespoons (45 ml) avocado oil, divided

2 teaspoons (12 g) kosher salt, divided

1 teaspoon (2 g) black pepper, divided

1 pound (450 g) salmon, cut into 4 fillets

3 tablespoons (45 ml) Clean Paleo Mayo (page 176)

½ pound (230 g) haricots verts

Butter lettuce or romaine hearts, for wrapping

½ cup (75 g) niçoise or kalamata olives, pitted and halved

½ cup (75 g) cherry tomatoes, halved

2 large hard-boiled eggs, quartered

¼ small red onion, thinly sliced

3 tablespoons (26 g) capers, drained

SAUCE

1 batch Clean Paleo Mayo (page 176)

3 anchovies packed in oil

½ lemon, juiced

2 cloves garlic

1 teaspoon (5 g) Dijon mustard

¼ teaspoon dried thyme

¼ teaspoon dried oregano

Kosher salt, to taste

Black pepper, to taste

Making a traditional salmon niçoise can be quite time-consuming. I've cut down significantly on the prep and cook time by doing everything on a baking sheet. This recipe comes together so beautifully when wrapped in lettuce leaves and finished off with a creamy, flavor-packed sauce. Don't shy away from the anchovies—their saltiness and subtle flavor really make these wraps sing. You're going to love this for lunch or as the centerpiece of a fabulous dinner party.

1 Preheat the oven to 375°F (190°C) and adjust the oven rack to the middle position. Line a baking sheet with parchment paper.

2 To make the salad, spread the potatoes onto the baking sheet and add 1½ tablespoons (22 ml) oil, 1 teaspoon (6 g) salt, and ½ teaspoon (1 g) pepper. Toss to evenly coat and bake for 20 minutes.

3 Sprinkle the salmon with ½ teaspoon (5 g) salt and ¼ teaspoon pepper. Coat it with the mayo. Drizzle the remaining 1½ tablespoons (22 ml) avocado oil onto the haricots verts and season with the remaining ½ teaspoon (5 g) salt and ¼ teaspoon pepper. Remove the potatoes from the oven and push them to one side of the baking sheet. Place the salmon in the center and the haricots verts on the other side. Bake until the salmon is cooked through and flakes easily with a fork, about 15 minutes. Let the salmon cool, then break up the pieces into large flakes.

4 Meanwhile, prepare the sauce. In a jar or medium bowl, add the mayo, anchovies, lemon juice, garlic, mustard, thyme, oregano, and a pinch of salt and pepper. Use an immersion blender to pulse until smooth and creamy throughout. Taste and adjust the salt and pepper, if necessary.

5 Assemble the wraps. Lay out the lettuce leaves and fill with the flaked salmon. Add the haricots verts, potatoes, olives, tomatoes, eggs, onion, and capers. Drizzle with the sauce and serve, eating them "taco style."

PREP TIME:
15 minutes

COOK TIME:
50 minutes

YIELD:
6 to 8 servings

chicken korma stew

CHICKEN

½ cup (125 g) coconut yogurt (see Notes)

1 tablespoon (15 ml) fresh lemon juice

½ teaspoon kosher salt

¼ teaspoon garam masala

¼ teaspoon coriander powder

¼ teaspoon turmeric powder

¼ teaspoon paprika

¼ teaspoon black pepper

2 pounds (900 g) boneless, skinless chicken thighs, patted dry

SAUCE

4 tablespoons (60 ml) ghee or grass-fed butter, divided

1 large yellow onion, diced

8 cloves garlic, minced

1 heaping teaspoon (2.7 g) minced fresh ginger

1 heaping teaspoon (2 g) garam masala

1 heaping teaspoon (2 g) coriander powder

Kosher salt, to taste

Black pepper, to taste

1 can (15 ounces [445 ml]) no-salt-added tomato sauce

1 red, yellow, or orange bell pepper, sliced

16 ounces (475 ml) full-fat canned coconut milk, plus more for serving (optional)

This authentic chicken korma is beyond delicious. What makes it feel so authentic to me is the inclusion of the garam masala. This is a blend of ground spices, originating from India, that is common across so many different cuisines. This fragrant stew pairs well with any type of rice, including cauliflower rice, or naan bread.

1   To make the chicken, in a shallow dish or resealable plastic bag, mix together the yogurt, lemon juice, salt, garam masala, coriander, turmeric, paprika, and pepper. Add the chicken, making sure it's submerged in the mixture, and set aside.

2   To make the sauce, melt 2 tablespoons (30 ml) of the ghee in a large pot or Dutch oven over medium heat. Add the onion and cook until completely dark golden-brown, 10 to 15 minutes. Be very careful not to burn it—stir frequently or lower the heat slightly if needed.

3   Add the garlic and ginger and sauté for 2 more minutes.

4   Stir in the garam masala, coriander, and a big pinch of salt and pepper. Let them bloom for a minute. Add your chicken mixture and briefly stir-fry to coat the chicken with the sauce.

5   Add the tomato sauce and bell pepper and cover the pot. Simmer for 15 minutes.

6   Add the coconut milk, mustard seed, and remaining 2 tablespoons (30 ml) ghee. Let it simmer uncovered for another 10 minutes. Taste it and add salt and black pepper, as needed.

½ teaspoon ground mustard
  seed
2 to 3 tablespoons (28 to
  43 g) arrowroot flour
2 to 3 tablespoons (30 to
  45 ml) filtered water
¼ cup (40 g) pine nuts,
  for garnish
Chopped cilantro, for garnish
2 lemons, cut into wedges

7 Make an arrowroot slurry by mixing the arrowroot with the water until smooth. Slowly pour a little at a time into the pot while stirring constantly. Keep adding until it reaches your desired thickness.

8 Divide the stew among bowls. Garnish with the pine nuts, cilantro, and extra coconut milk, if you'd like. Top off with a nice squeeze of lemon juice.

NOTES:

If you're able to have cow's milk, feel free to use regular yogurt instead.

If you can find it, substitute powdered fenugreek for the mustard seed. This herb, native to India and the Mediterranean, has a subtle maple syrup flavor.

You can dice up your chicken after it has cooked or leave it as is. It'll be so soft, I wouldn't worry too much about it.

PREP TIME:
10 minutes +
chill time

COOK TIME:
N/A

YIELD:
4 to 6 servings

waldorf tuna salad

3 cans (5 ounces [141 g])
wild-caught tuna, drained

¾ cup (110 g) red grapes,
halved

⅔ cup (100 g) pecans,
chopped

1 medium green apple, diced

¼ yellow onion, diced

⅓ cup (50 g) diced celery

⅓ to ½ cup (80 to 120 ml)
Clean Paleo Mayo
(page 176)

½ lemon, juiced

½ to ¾ teaspoon kosher salt

¼ teaspoon garlic powder

Black pepper, to taste

There's something about mixing fruit into savory salads that really puts a smile on my face. I knew this Waldorf tuna salad was something special when I set the leftovers in the refrigerator at night and saw they had disappeared by morning. My husband, Tim, said to me, "That was really good. Sorry I ate it all." Humph. (This is basically the story of my life.) We love the combination of apple, grapes, and pecans with the tuna. It's so creamy, crunchy, and delicious!

1 In a large bowl, toss together the tuna, grapes, pecans, apple, onion, celery, mayo, lemon juice, salt, garlic powder, and a pinch of black pepper. Taste for additional seasoning. You may need 1 tablespoon (15 ml) more or less of mayo, depending on your preference. Refrigerate the salad for 1 to 2 hours before serving.

PREP TIME:
5 minutes

COOK TIME:
40 minutes

YIELD:
6 to 8 servings

tom kha soup

3 cans (13.5 ounces [395 ml]) full-fat coconut milk

1 quart (1 L) chicken bone broth or low-sodium chicken broth (see Notes)

6 to 8 Thai chiles, depending on heat preferences (see Notes)

1½-inch (3.75 cm) knob fresh ginger, peeled and minced

8 ounces (230 g) cremini or baby bella mushrooms, thinly sliced

2 pounds (900 g) large shrimp, peeled and deveined

2 limes, juiced

2½ tablespoons (37 ml) fish sauce

2½ tablespoons (37 ml) coconut aminos

Kosher salt, to taste

Black pepper, to taste

Coarsely chopped fresh cilantro, for serving

Lime wedges, for serving

Tom kha is a flavorful Thai soup that is spicy and sour and made with a coconut milk base. It takes very little time to prep, and you can dump everything into one pot, which is a huge bonus! You're going to love this tangy, salty soup full of delectable shrimp. Don't skimp on those Thai chiles, as they infuse a ton of flavor and fabulous heat! Serve it by itself or pour over rice or cauliflower rice.

1 In a large pot or Dutch oven, bring the coconut milk and broth to a boil over medium-high heat. Lower the heat to medium and add the Thai chiles and ginger. Simmer for 10 minutes.

2 Add the mushrooms and simmer, stirring occasionally, for 5 minutes.

3 Add the shrimp, lime juice, fish sauce, and coconut aminos. Simmer until the shrimp are cooked through, about 5 minutes.

4 Taste and add more Thai chiles if it is not spicy enough for you. Continue simmering for another 10 minutes.

5 Check for seasoning, adding salt and black pepper if necessary. Add even more Thai chiles, if you'd like.

6 Top off the soup with chopped cilantro and serve with fresh lime wedges.

NOTES:

I recommend using bone broth if you have access to it. However, chicken broth is a fine substitute.

Taste the soup regularly and add more Thai chiles if the soup isn't spicy enough for you. I end up using a large handful!

PREP TIME:
15 minutes +
cashew soak time

COOK TIME:
40 minutes

YIELD:
8 servings

low—carb cheeseburger soup

1½ cups (225 g) raw
  cashews
6 strips bacon, diced
2 pounds (900 g) grass-fed
  90/10 ground beef
2½ cups (595 ml) beef
  bone broth
1 can (13.5 ounces
  [395 ml]) full-fat
  coconut milk
1 can (6 ounces [180 g])
  tomato paste
2 teaspoons (12 g)
  kosher salt
1½ pounds (680 g)
  broccoli florets
Black pepper, to taste
Sliced avocado, for garnish
Fresh parsley, for garnish

If I told you you could have all the fabulous flavors of a cheeseburger in a nutritious and dairy-free soup, would you believe me? Well, this creamy cheeseburger soup is made rich with cashews, bacon, and bone broth. It also has plenty of broccoli because we all need our vegetables, don't we? You're going to love this so much, you won't even miss the cheese (or the bun!).

1 Add the cashews to a bowl and cover with boiling water. Let sit, uncovered, for 1½ hours. Drain the soaked cashews and rinse well with cold water. Set aside.

2 In a large pot, cook the bacon pieces over medium heat until crispy, 3 to 4 minutes. Increase the heat to medium-high and add the ground beef. Cook, stirring often to break the beef apart into even pieces, until it is brown throughout, 8 to 10 minutes.

3 Meanwhile, in the pitcher of a high-speed blender, add the broth, coconut milk, tomato paste, drained cashews, and salt. Blend on high speed until smooth and creamy throughout.

4 Transfer the cashew mixture to the pot and stir well. Bring to a boil over medium-high heat, stirring occasionally.

5 Reduce the heat to a simmer, add the broccoli florets, and cook until the broccoli is fork-tender, another 10 to 15 minutes. Taste for seasoning (salt and pepper) and remove from the heat. Serve topped with avocado and parsley—or your preferred cheeseburger toppings!

PREP TIME:
30 minutes

COOK TIME:
N/A

YIELD:
8 servings

DAIRY

antipasti salad

- 8 ounces (230 g) Genoa salami, sliced (see Note)
- 8 ounces (230 g) Soppressata, sliced (see Note)
- 8 ounces (230 g) white cheddar, cut into bite-size chunks
- 8 ounces (230 g) fresh mozzarella, cut into bite-size chunks
- 1½ cups (225 g) cherry tomatoes, halved
- 1 can (14 ounces [396 g]) artichoke hearts in water, drained and sliced
- ½ cup (75 g) sliced roasted red peppers
- 2 tablespoons (30 ml) juice from the red pepper jar
- ½ cup (75 g) pitted kalamata olives, chopped
- ⅓ cup (50 g) green olives, pitted and chopped
- 1½ tablespoons (22 ml) extra virgin olive oil
- 3 tablespoons (45 ml) red wine vinegar
- ½ teaspoon black pepper
- ¼ cup (6 g) basil leaves, coarsely chopped

NOTE:

Read the labels on the Soppressata and salami for added sugar and fillers.

Stop defaulting to a meat and cheese platter when you entertain. Instead, wow your guests and make them smile with this antipasti "salad" that's full of different types of salami, cheese, and accompaniments. A bit of tang from red wine vinegar and a fresh hint of basil tie everything together!

1 In a large serving bowl, toss together the Genoa salami, and Soppressata, cheddar, mozzarella, tomatoes, artichokes, red peppers, and the pepper juice.

2 Mix in the black and green olives. Drizzle the olive oil over the entire dish, followed by the vinegar and black pepper.

3 Mix thoroughly and add the basil right before serving.

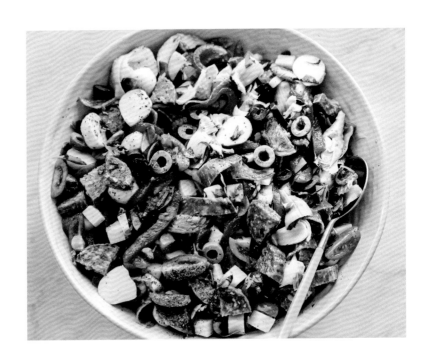

PREP TIME:
15 minutes +
cashew soak time

COOK TIME:
N/A

YIELD:
6 to 8 servings

DAIRY

greek salad with cashew tzatziki

DRESSING

1½ cups (225 g) raw cashews

1 cup (240 ml) filtered water

2 tablespoons (30 ml) fresh
lemon juice

5 cloves garlic

1 tablespoon (15 ml)
white vinegar (distilled
or white wine)

¾ teaspoon kosher salt, plus
more to taste

1½ cups (225 g) grated
English cucumber (about
1 large cucumber)

2 heaping tablespoons (8 g)
fresh dill, chopped, plus
more for serving (optional)

Black pepper, to taste

SALAD

6 Persian cucumbers, halved,
seeded, and sliced

1½ cups (225 g) cherry
tomatoes, halved

2 green bell peppers, diced

1 white onion, thinly sliced

1 cup (150 g) pitted kalamata
olives

2½ tablespoons (25 g)
capers, drained, plus more
for serving (optional)

2 tablespoons (8 g) dried
oregano

6 ounces (169 g) sheep's milk
feta cheese, crumbled
(omit for Clean Paleo)

Kosher salt, to taste

Black pepper, to taste

This refreshing Greek salad is made with sliced cucumbers instead of lettuce for its base. It includes tons of fresh vegetables and snappy capers and olives. The cashew-based, Clean Paleo tzatziki hits all the right notes and will leave you licking your bowl clean. The flavors develop more the longer it sits, so leftovers are even more amazing!

1. To make the dressing, add the cashews to a bowl and cover with boiling water. Let sit, uncovered, for 1½ hours. Drain thoroughly and rinse well with cold water. Set aside.

2. In the pitcher of a high-speed blender, add the water, lemon juice, garlic, vinegar, salt, and cashews. Blend on high speed, scraping down the sides as necessary. You want it to be thick and creamy throughout.

3. Add the cucumber and blend until completely incorporated.

4. Transfer to a bowl and stir in the dill and pepper. Taste and adjust for salt and pepper. Refrigerate to allow it to thicken.

5. When you're ready to make the salad, toss together the cucumbers, tomatoes, bell peppers, onion, olives, capers, oregano, and feta (if using) in a large bowl. Sprinkle with a large pinch of salt and black pepper.

6. Add your desired amount of tzatziki dressing, tossing to combine. You will most likely have plenty of dressing left over, which you can store in an airtight container in the refrigerator for up to 5 days.

7. Serve right away, garnished with extra capers and fresh dill, if desired.

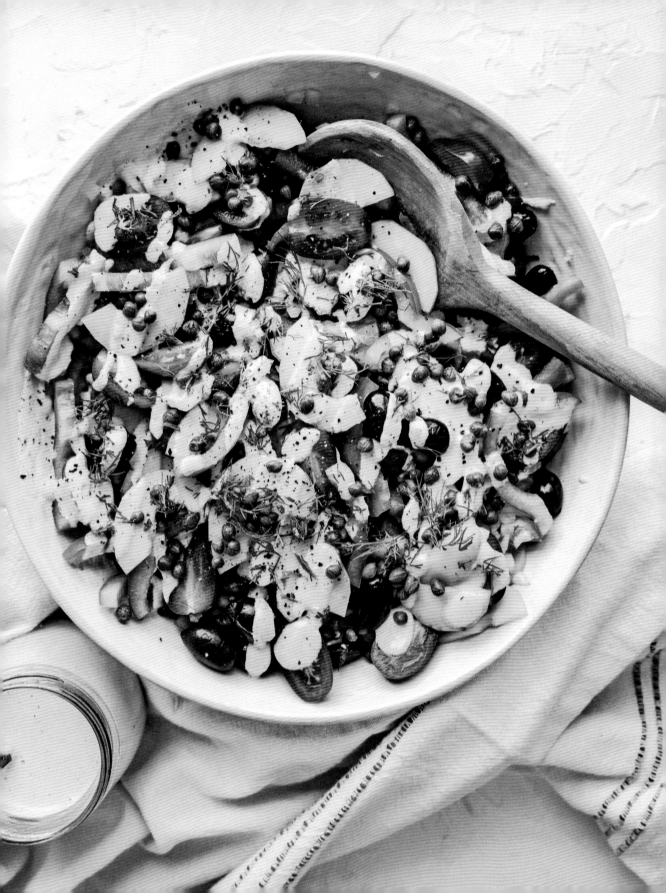

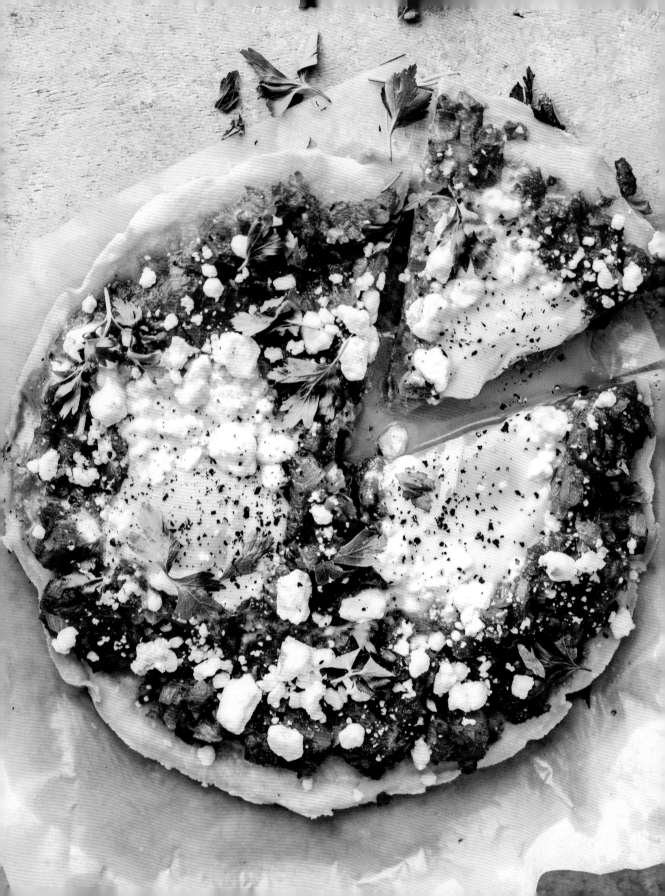

apps, entertaining & finger food

THERE'S SOMETHING TO BE SAID about creating a really beautiful spread when you are hosting a gathering at your house. The same can be true about attending a big party and being asked to bring an awesome dish that everyone can grab and enjoy. I created this chapter in the hopes of being able to appeal to a wide variety of people with dishes that are exciting, delicious, and won't take all day to prepare.

Here, you'll find Chicken Liver Pâté that will win over anyone—even those who don't like liver. You'll also find fried calamari with a tomato-garlic dipping sauce that's so good it will make you forget about ever ordering calamari at a restaurant again. Not to mention the Moroccan Chicken Wings and an insanely delectable Shakshuka Pizza.

You're going to be overwhelmed by how much goodness is here. In fact, I urge you to call all your favorite people and invite them over. Don't blame me, though, if they won't leave.

◀ Shakshuka Pizza, page 60

PREP TIME:
20 minutes

COOK TIME:
22 minutes

YIELD:
2 or 3 servings

SWEETENER / DAIRY

shakshuka pizza

CRUST
½ cup (120 ml) full-fat canned coconut milk
¼ cup (60 ml) ghee
1 cup (120 g) tapioca flour
¼ cup (30 g) coconut flour
1 teaspoon (6 g) kosher salt
1 large egg, lightly beaten

TOPPING
2 tablespoons (30 ml) ghee or extra-virgin olive oil, plus more for drizzling
1 small yellow onion, diced
2 cloves garlic, minced
2 teaspoons (6 g) coconut sugar
1 teaspoon (15 g) harissa paste
1 teaspoon (2.5 g) ground cumin
½ teaspoon ground basil
Kosher salt, to taste
Black pepper, to taste
1 can (14.5 ounces [410 g]) diced tomatoes
1 tablespoon (16 g) tomato paste
2 or 3 large eggs (see Notes)
4 ounces (113 g) goat cheese (see Notes)
Handful chopped parsley, for garnish

Shakshuka is a Mediterranean breakfast dish of eggs poached in a sauce of tomatoes, chile peppers, and onions, often spiced with a bit of cumin. Transforming it into a pizza dish, with eggs baked right on top, was genius, if I do say so myself. Harissa is a fabulous hot chile pepper paste that can usually be found in the ethnic foods section of the grocery store.

1 Preheat the oven to 450°F (230°C). Place a 12-inch (30 cm) cast-iron skillet into the oven to heat up. After 10 minutes, remove the skillet from the oven and set aside.

2 To make the crust, in a small saucepan over medium-low heat, combine the coconut milk and ghee until they begin to simmer, about 3 minutes. Remove from the heat.

3 In a large bowl, sift together the tapioca flour, coconut flour, and salt. Pour the coconut milk mixture on top. Mix until thoroughly combined (I used my hands to do this). Let the mixture sit for a couple of minutes to allow the flours to fully absorb the liquid. Add the beaten egg and mix again with your hands until everything is well combined.

4 Carefully cover the cast-iron skillet with unbleached parchment paper and pour the crust mixture into the middle. Using a small spatula or the back of a spoon, spread the mixture until it covers the base of the skillet.

5 Bake until the edges begin to crisp up, 12 to 15 minutes. Remove from the oven and turn down the heat to 375°F (190°C).

6 Meanwhile, prepare the topping. Heat the ghee or oil in a medium saucepan over medium heat and add the onion. Cook until soft and translucent, 5 to 7 minutes. Add the garlic, coconut sugar, harissa, cumin, basil, a pinch of salt, and a few twists of black pepper. Cook

for an additional minute. Add the tomatoes and tomato paste and simmer, stirring occasionally, until the flavors have married, about 15 minutes. Remove from the heat.

7   Top the pizza crust with half the tomato sauce, leaving about 1 inch (2.5 cm) around the border. Create 2 or 3 wells on top to hold the eggs. Carefully crack an egg into each well. Sprinkle each with the goat cheese.

8   Bake until the egg whites have set, but the yolks are runny, and the crust has browned, 7 to 10 minutes.

9   Serve immediately, garnished with a few sprinkles of fresh parsley and a drizzle of olive oil.

PREP TIME:
10 minutes
COOK TIME:
40 minutes
YIELD:
4 to 6 servings

SWEETENER

WINGS
2½ pounds (1.13 kg) chicken drumettes or wings
2 tablespoons (30 ml) avocado oil
1 teaspoon (6 g) kosher salt
½ teaspoon black pepper

SAUCE
¼ cup (60 ml) coconut aminos
¼ cup (60 ml) dry sherry
2 tablespoons (30 ml) avocado oil
2 tablespoons (30 ml) fresh lemon juice
2 tablespoons (30 ml) honey
4 cloves garlic, pressed
1 teaspoon (2 g) curry powder
½ teaspoon dried thyme
¼ teaspoon dried oregano
¼ teaspoon dried ginger
¼ teaspoon black pepper
1½ tablespoons (12 g) arrowroot flour
1½ tablespoons (22 ml) filtered water
⅓ cup (50 g) thinly sliced scallions, for garnish

moroccan chicken wings

The flavor of these wings is going to blow your dang mind. The Moroccan flavors I've infused into the wing sauce are just exquisite. You're going to want to serve these at any and all get-togethers. Or heck, do like I do and pair them with a big, juicy salad. Mm, mmm.

1 Preheat the oven to 400°F (200°C) and adjust the oven rack to the middle position. Line a baking sheet with aluminum foil and top with a wire rack.

2 To make the wings, on a large cutting board, spread out the chicken in a single layer, skin side up. Using a paper towel, pat the skin as dry as you can.

3 Transfer the chicken to a large bowl. Add the oil, salt, and pepper. Toss to thoroughly coat.

4 Place the chicken on the wire rack. Make sure no chicken is touching. (If they are too close, they won't crisp.) Bake for 35 minutes. Turn the oven to a low broil and cook until crisp and golden, 5 minutes more.

5 Meanwhile, prepare the sauce. In a small saucepan, whisk together the coconut aminos, sherry, oil, lemon juice, honey, garlic, curry, thyme, oregano, ginger, and pepper. Cook over medium heat until it reaches a low boil. Turn down the heat to low and simmer for 15 to 20 minutes, stirring occasionally.

6 While the sauce is cooking, prepare an arrowroot slurry by combing the arrowroot flour with the water in a small bowl until smooth. During the last few minutes of sauce cook time, continue whisking while slowly pouring in enough slurry to reach your desired consistency.

7 When the wings are done, transfer them to a large bowl. Pour the sauce on top, mix, sprinkle with the scallions, and serve.

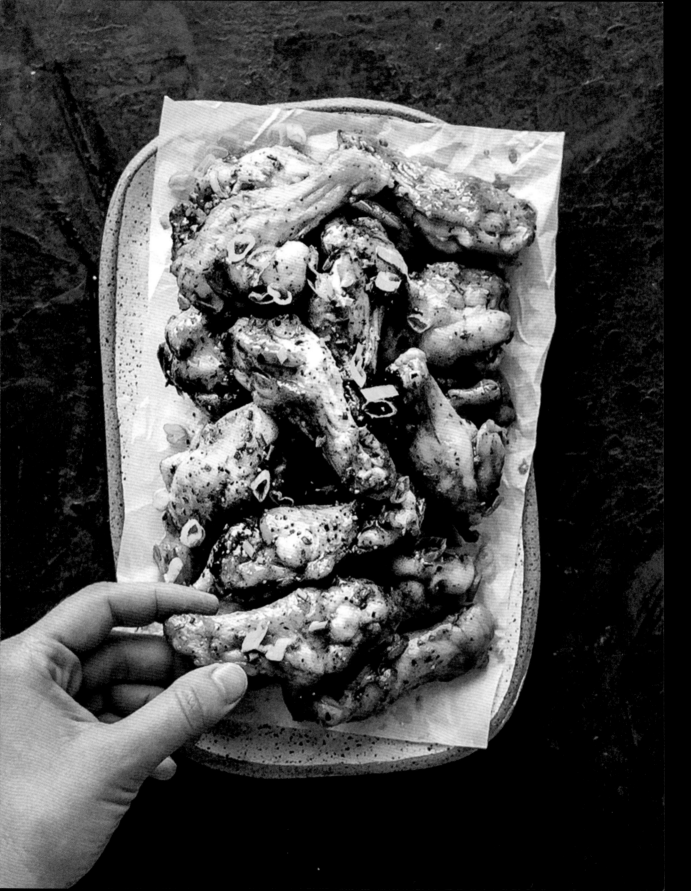

PREP TIME:
10 minutes
COOK TIME:
5 minutes
YIELD:
1½ cups (340 g)

LEGUMES

bone broth hummus

1 can (15 ounces [439 g]) chickpeas, drained, rinsed, and skins removed
½ cup (120 ml) beef or chicken bone broth
1 large lemon, juiced
¼ cup (56 g) creamy tahini, well stirred
2½ to 3 tablespoons (37 to 45 ml) olive oil or avocado oil
2 large cloves garlic
½ teaspoon ground cumin
1 teaspoon (6 g) kosher salt, plus more to taste
Black pepper, to taste

I am pretty sure that incorporating bone broth into my home-made dips and hummus is my favorite thing to do. It adds so much protein, flavor, and goodness that I can't resist. This hummus will become a staple in your refrigerator's snack drawer or one of the quickest and tastiest things you can bring to any potluck or get-together.

1   Combine the chickpeas in a saucepan with the bone broth. Bring to a simmer over medium-low heat and cook until the majority of the broth has been absorbed by the chickpeas, 3 to 5 minutes.

2   Transfer the mixture to a food processor or high-speed blender. Add the lemon juice, tahini, oil, garlic, cumin, and salt.

3   Process until smooth and creamy throughout, adding a tiny bit of oil as needed to smooth out completely.

4   Taste for additional salt and pepper, if you'd like.

5   Store in the refrigerator in an airtight container for up to 1 week.

PREP TIME:
5 minutes
COOK TIME:
15 minutes
YIELD:
1½ cups (340 g)

chicken liver pâté

1 pound (450 g) organic chicken livers

⅓ cup (80 ml) ghee or grass-fed butter, divided

2 medium shallots, finely chopped

6 cloves garlic, minced (see Note)

2 teaspoons (2.8 g) ground bay leaves

Kosher salt, to taste (see Note)

Black pepper, to taste

2 tablespoons (8 g) fresh parsley leaves, chopped

2 tablespoons (30 ml) apple cider vinegar

1 tablespoon (7 g) ground cumin

1½ teaspoons (3.5 g) smoked paprika

1 large hard-boiled egg

NOTE:

To make this baby friendly (if under one year old), simply omit the salt and garlic.

I know what you're thinking, but let me stop you right there. This was one of the very first recipes I fed to my daughter, Sophie, when she was six months old and ready to start solid foods. She would eat this stuff straight from the spoon. My husband says this recipe is warm, comforting, and barely tastes like liver, which sounds like a win to me. Serve it with your favorite cut veggies and sliced green apple at your next gathering and see how many of your friends and family you can get on board!

1 Put the chicken livers into a colander and rinse with cold water a few times, since they will most likely be very bloody. Pat dry and set aside.

2 Melt 1 tablespoon (15 ml) the ghee in a large frying pan or cast-iron skillet over medium heat. Add the shallots, garlic (if using), and bay leaves with a few sprinkles of salt (if using) and pepper. Sauté until the shallots are translucent, 3 to 4 minutes.

3 Add the livers. Sauté for another 4 to 5 minutes, then add the parsley, vinegar, cumin, and paprika. Use tongs and continue mixing the livers and cooking them for another 4 to 5 minutes. You will want all (or at least most) of the vinegar to evaporate.

4 Transfer the mixture to the bowl of a food processor. Slowly pulse the livers, adding the remaining ghee, 1 tablespoon (15 ml) at a time. Add in the egg and pulse again. Once everything has been incorporated, pulse the pâté until it is nice and smooth.

5 Taste your mixture and add any salt or pepper to your preference.

6 Serve at room temperature. This will keep in the refrigerator in an airtight container for up to 1 week. To serve another day, pull it out and let it sit at room temperature for about an hour and give it a nice stir before serving.

PREP TIME:
15 minutes

COOK TIME:
10 minutes

YIELD:
4 servings

calamari with tomato-garlic aioli

1 pound (450 g) wild-caught squid tubes (see Notes)

1 cup (120 g) arrowroot flour

½ cup (60 g) macadamia nuts, finely crushed (see Notes)

1 tablespoon (18 g) kosher salt

Coconut oil, for frying

Chopped fresh parsley, for garnish

1 batch Tomato-Garlic Aioli (page 182), for serving

Fresh lemon wedges, for serving

You're going to be ecstatic when you see how simple it is to make delicious calamari at home. The Tomato-Garlic Aioli from chapter 9 is the perfect pairing, as it's rich and creamy and complements the crispy squid just wonderfully. Definitely use this dish to impress.

1 Slice the squid into rings about ½ inch (13 mm) thick and pat as dry as possible.

2 In a large bowl, combine the arrowroot flour, nuts, and salt.

3 In a large saucepan over medium-high heat, heat about 2 inches (5 cm) of coconut oil for a few minutes until it begins to slightly bubble but is not smoking.

4 Add the calamari rings to the flour/nut mixture, making sure they are coated completely. Place them on a parchment-lined baking sheet and set the sheet next to the stove as a launching pad for the calamari to go into the oil.

5 Carefully transfer the calamari into the oil without overcrowding; you'll need to do this in batches. Watch them carefully and pull them out of the oil between 3 and 5 minutes, when they seem to look crisp throughout. Use a slotted spoon or spider to pull them out carefully, and lay them out on paper towels to slightly drain. Adjust the heat in between batches if the oil starts to smoke.

6 Serve hot, sprinkled with the parsley, along with the Tomato-Garlic Aioli and lemon wedges.

NOTES:

You can buy squid tubes and slice them into pieces on your own or you can find already cut calamari rings. You will find them in the frozen fish area, at the seafood counter, and in Asian markets as well.

I prefer to use a mallet or rolling pin to really crush my macadamia nuts into fine pieces.

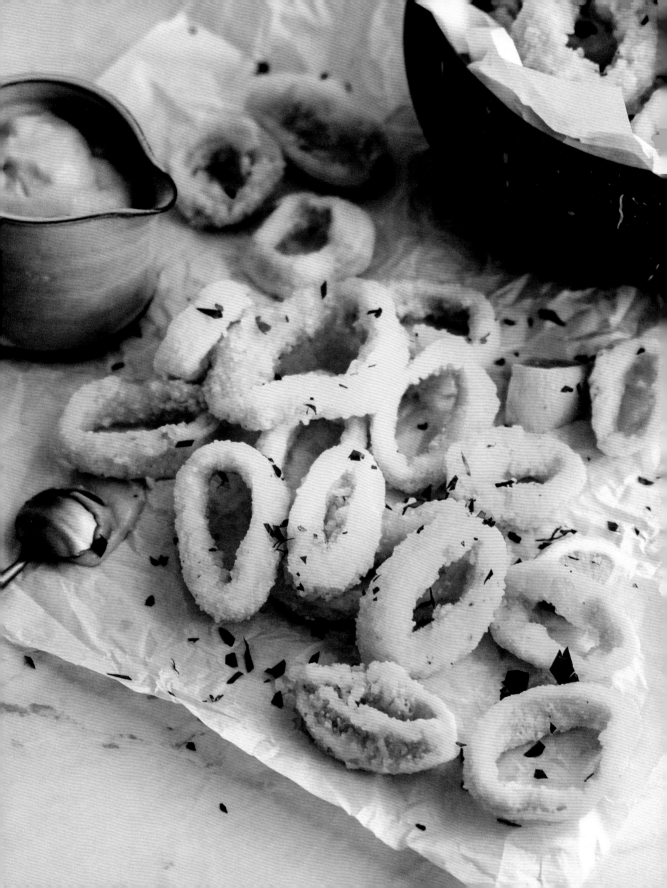

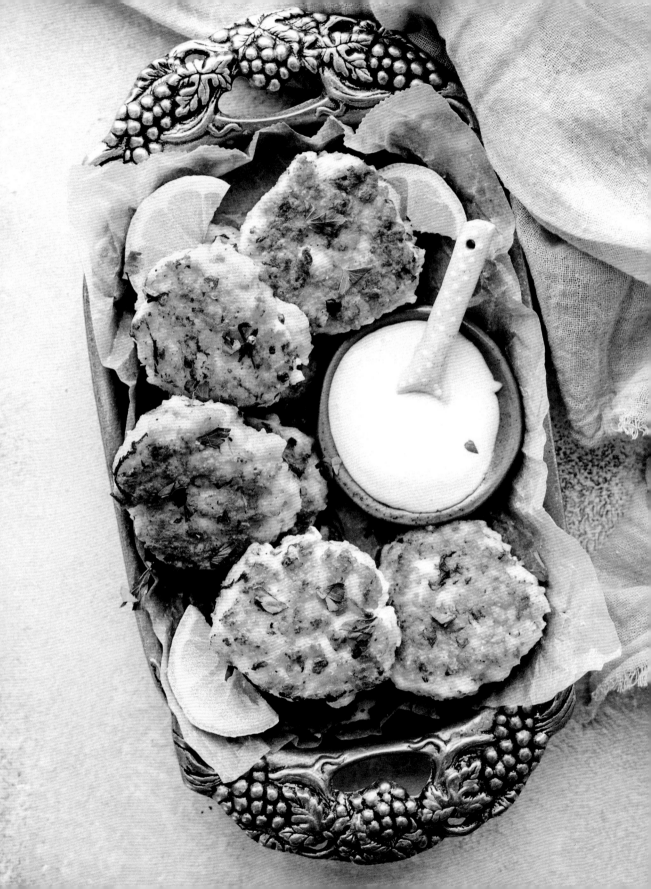

PREP TIME:
15 minutes

COOK TIME:
20 minutes

YIELD:
4 servings

DAIRY

shrimp cakes with lemon aioli

SHRIMP CAKES

1 pound (450 g) large shrimp, peeled, deveined, and patted dry

4 ounces (113 g) Parmesan cheese, grated

1 large egg

3 tablespoons (45 ml) Clean Paleo Mayo (page 176)

3 tablespoons (7.5 g) finely chopped basil, plus more for serving (optional)

½ teaspoon kosher salt

¼ teaspoon black pepper

5 tablespoons (30 g) almond flour

1 tablespoon (8 g) arrowroot flour

2 tablespoons (30 ml) avocado oil or ghee

LEMON AIOLI

½ cup (120 ml) Clean Paleo Mayo (page 176)

2 tablespoons (30 ml) fresh lemon juice

3 cloves garlic, coarsely chopped

1 teaspoon (2 g) lemon zest

These little cakes make for the perfect hors d'oeuvres for any get-together. The basil and Parmesan cheese inside really take them over the top. The cakes come together very quickly, and the lemony aioli on the side is just the right accompaniment. I've even topped off some awesome salads with these shrimp cakes. You can thin out the lemon aioli with some water and turn it into a dressing. Voilà!

1 To make the shrimp cakes, chop the shrimp into ¼-inch (6 mm) pieces and transfer to a large bowl.

2 Add the Parmesan, egg, mayo, basil, salt, and pepper. Stir together and add the almond and arrowroot flours. Mix until the batter is well combined and the flours are evenly dispersed.

3 Heat a large nonstick skillet over medium heat and add the oil. Using a level ice cream scoop, add cakes to the pan, leaving about 1½ inches (4 cm) of space between them. Lightly flatten the tops until they are about ½ inch (13 mm) thick. Cook until golden brown, 4 to 5 minutes. Flip carefully and cook until browned, another 3 to 4 minutes. Transfer to a paper towel–lined plate or cutting board.

4 Meanwhile, make the aioli. Combine the mayo, lemon juice, garlic, and zest in a glass jar. Blend using an immersion blender until smooth and creamy throughout.

5 Serve the shrimp cakes hot with the aioli and extra chopped basil, if desired.

NOTE:

The Lemon Aioli makes a great dip on its own!

PREP TIME:
10 minutes
COOK TIME:
30 minutes
YIELD:
6 to 8 servings

pumpkin alfredo poutine

FRENCH FRIES
4 large sweet potatoes, peeled
Ghee or coconut oil, melted, for mixing
2 tablespoons (15 g) tapioca flour or starch
1½ teaspoons (9 g) kosher salt

PUMPKIN ALFREDO
¼ cup (60 g) ghee or grass-fed butter
½ cup (75 g) diced yellow onion
2 cups (475 ml) full-fat canned coconut milk or heavy cream
½ cup (120 g) canned pumpkin puree
1 teaspoon (3 g) minced garlic
1 teaspoon (2 g) white pepper
1 teaspoon (3 g) garlic powder
2 tablespoons (16 g) arrowroot flour
Kosher salt, to taste
¼ cup (40 g) finely chopped fresh chives, for garnish
Goat cheese crumbles, for garnish

The first time I tried poutine was just a few years ago as a midnight snack at a Canadian wedding. Boy, was my world turned upside down in the best way possible. French fries, cheese curds, and gravy? To say I was impressed is an understatement. I knew I had to recreate this tasty snack as soon as I was home, and since this was a fall wedding, the first thing I thought to incorporate into my rendition of poutine was sweet potatoes. No need to be too light-handed with the chives and crumbled goat cheese. The toppings really bring this dish completely over the top!

1   Preheat the oven to 425°F (220°C) and adjust the oven rack to the middle position. (If two baking sheets won't fit side by side, then adjust two racks to the upper and lower thirds.)

2   To make the fries, cut the sweet potatoes into fry-shaped pieces, about 1 inch (2.5 cm) thick. Try to cut them into similar-size pieces so the fries will bake evenly.

3   Toss the potatoes into a mixing bowl and add just enough ghee to coat. Add the tapioca flour and salt. Mix or shake to distribute evenly (there shouldn't be any "powdery" spots).

4   Pour the fries directly onto two dark, nonstick baking sheets. (Note: Lining the baking sheets with aluminum foil or parchment paper can lead to mixed results!) Arrange the fries in a single layer with a little space between each. They need space to crisp up! Bake for 15 minutes and flip the fries over to cook both sides. If your baking sheets are on two separate racks, switch their positions now.

5   Bake until the fries look crispy around the edges, another 10 to 15 minutes.

6   While the fries are finishing up in the oven, prepare the pumpkin alfredo. Melt the ghee or butter in a medium saucepan over medium heat. Add the onion and cook until translucent, 4 to 5 minutes.

7   Add the coconut milk or heavy cream and whisk until well combined.

8   Mix in the pumpkin, garlic, pepper, and garlic powder, whisking over medium heat until it reaches a low boil.

9   Lower the heat to a simmer and whisk in the arrowroot flour, stirring until it reaches a thick, alfredo-like consistency.

10 Once the arrowroot powder has been absorbed, and your sauce is looking relatively smooth (with the exception of the onion), remove it from the heat.

11 Carefully transfer the pumpkin alfredo to a blender (or use an immersion blender) and puree until everything is well incorporated and perfectly smooth, 15 to 20 seconds. Taste and add salt, if necessary.

12 Arrange the fries on a large platter or plate. Pour the pumpkin alfredo on top and garnish with the chives and goat cheese. Use tongs for serving.

13 Store any leftover pumpkin alfredo in an airtight container for up to 1 week in the refrigerator.

creamy cashew ranch dip

PREP TIME:
5 minutes +
cashew soak time

COOK TIME:
N/A

YIELD:
about 1 cup (220 ml)

1½ cups (225 g) raw cashews
⅓ cup (80 ml) chicken bone broth
⅓ cup (80 ml) filtered water
2 tablespoons (30 ml) fresh lemon juice
1 tablespoon (15 ml) coconut oil
1 tablespoon (8.5 g) nutritional yeast
1¼ teaspoons (3.8 g) garlic powder
½ teaspoon dried dill
Kosher salt, to taste
Black pepper, to taste

If you're looking for a tasty dip that will pair well with both cut veggies and chips, then look no further. Ranch dip is always a crowd favorite, and I'm always sure to bring it to a potluck or dinner party. This dip is satisfying without being too heavy.

1   Place the cashews in a bowl and cover with boiling water. Set aside for 1½ hours. Drain and rinse well with cold water. Let drain thoroughly.

2   Transfer the cashews to the pitcher of a high-speed blender and add the broth, water, lemon juice, oil, nutritional yeast, garlic powder, dill, and a pinch of salt and pepper. Blend on high speed until it looks smooth and creamy. Depending on what type of blender you have, you may need to scrape down the sides a few times. Taste for salt and pepper.

3   Store in an airtight container in the refrigerator for up to 1 week.

PREP TIME:
10 minutes +
cashew soak time

COOK TIME:
30 minutes

YIELD:
6 servings

spinach artichoke dip

1½ cups (225 g) raw cashews

¾ cup (180 ml) vegetable broth

¾ cup (180 ml) coconut cream (see Note)

¼ cup (15 g) nutritional yeast

1 lemon, juiced

1 teaspoon (6 g) kosher salt

1½ tablespoons (22 ml) avocado oil or coconut oil

1 shallot, sliced

8 cloves garlic, minced

2 cans (14 ounces [394 g]) artichoke hearts in water, drained

4 cups (141 g) loosely packed fresh spinach

NOTE:

Coconut cream is the cream that has separated and risen to the top of a can of full-fat coconut milk that has been refrigerated overnight. Alternatively, use cans of coconut cream, available in the ethnic foods section at the grocery store. Make sure it has at least 10 to 12 grams of fat for a super creamy and luscious dip.

This easy spinach artichoke dip is made with raw cashews, fresh spinach, coconut cream, and plenty of love. It's kid approved, and it pairs wonderfully with cut-up veggies, gluten-free bread, or other snacks. It's the perfect dip to have at a get-together, as it keeps well outside of the refrigerator, too!

1 Add the cashews to a bowl and cover with boiling water. Let sit, uncovered, for 1½ hours. Rinse and drain thoroughly.

2 Preheat the oven to 425°F (220°C) and adjust the oven rack to the middle position.

3 Transfer the cashews to a high-speed blender or food processor. Add the broth, coconut cream, nutritional yeast, lemon juice, and salt. Blend on high speed until smooth and creamy throughout, 1 to 2 minutes. You may need to scrape down the sides a few times or use a tamper.

4 In a medium skillet over medium-low heat, warm the oil. Once it is hot (about 1 minute), add the shallot and garlic. Sauté until fragrant and soft, stirring frequently, 2 to 3 minutes. Transfer the mixture to the blender.

5 Add the artichokes to the blender, along with the spinach. Pulse a few times or blend just until broken down a little bit. You want the mixture to be chunky, not smooth.

6 Transfer to a 2-quart (2 L) baking dish. Bake until the edges begin to turn golden brown, 22 to 26 minutes. You can turn the broiler on low at the end for a few minutes to speed up this process, too. Serve warm.

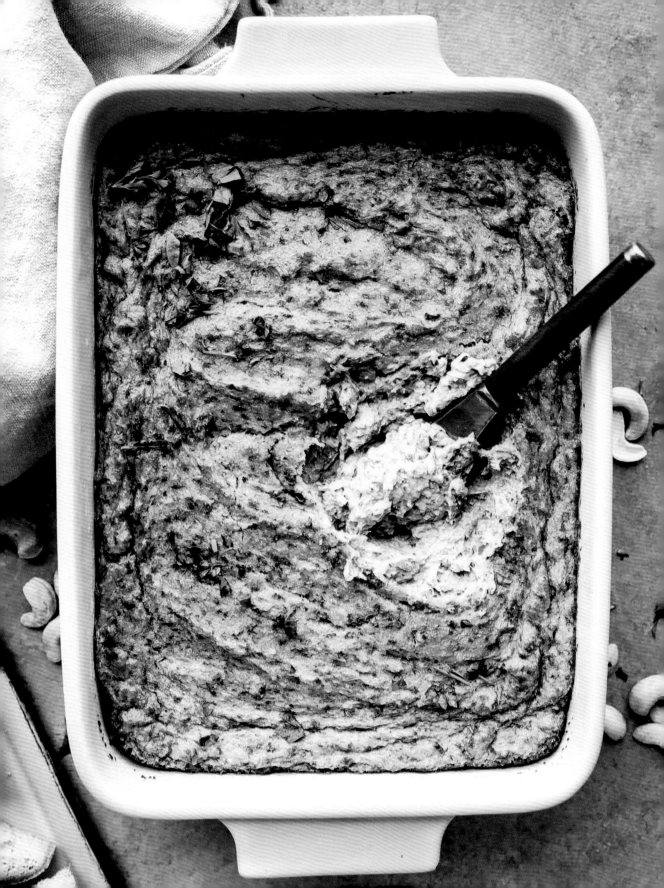

PREP TIME:
20 minutes

COOK TIME:
50 minutes

YIELD:
4 to 6 servings

SWEETENER / DAIRY

caramelized onion and blueberry tart

CARAMELIZED ONIONS
2½ tablespoons (37 ml) ghee or coconut oil
½ large red onion, sliced
½ large yellow onion, sliced
1 tablespoon (9 g) coconut sugar

CRUST
½ cup (120 ml) full-fat canned coconut milk
¼ cup (60 ml) ghee or coconut oil, plus more for the pan
1 cup (120 g) tapioca flour
¼ cup (30 g) coconut flour
1 teaspoon (6 g) kosher salt
1 large egg, lightly beaten

BLUEBERRY PRESERVES
2 tablespoons (19 g) grass-fed gelatin (see Note)
1 lemon, juiced
1 tablespoon (15 ml) coconut oil
3 cups (450 g) blueberries, divided
2 tablespoons (30 ml) raw honey or pure maple syrup
Pinch of kosher salt

2 to 4 ounces (56 to 113 g) soft goat cheese, for sprinkling on top
Sliced fresh basil, for garnish

Caramelized onions are the best addition to my morning eggs, on top of a burger, or—in this case—as the base for this perfectly savory and sweet tart. This beauty would be a wonderful centerpiece for a weekend brunch. If you'd like, you can add meat topping to it—sliced lamb or beef go very well with the blueberry preserves and caramelized onions. I knew this savory-meets-sweet tart was the ticket as soon as I saw the empty pan on the counter just a few hours after baking it!

1   To make the caramelized the onions, heat a large skillet over medium-high heat for 2 minutes. Add the 2½ tablespoons (37 ml) ghee or coconut oil. When melted, add the onions and cook until they become soft and begin to turn brown, 8 to 10 minutes, stirring frequently. Reduce the heat to low and continue cooking the onions for another 15 minutes, stirring frequently. They will be completely brown and may begin to stick to the pan. That is a good thing, just be sure to stir so they do not burn. Sprinkle with the coconut sugar and cook for another minute. Remove from the heat.

2   Meanwhile, make the crust. Preheat the oven to 425°F (220°C) and adjust the oven rack to the middle position. Place an 11-inch (28 cm) tart pan or 14 x 5-inch (36 x 13-cm) rectangular tart pan on the counter and lightly grease with oil.

3   In a small saucepan over medium-low heat, warm the coconut milk and ¼ cup (60 ml) ghee until they begin to simmer, 2 to 3 minutes.

4   Sift together the tapioca flour, coconut flour, and salt into a large bowl. Pour the coconut milk mixture on top and mix until thoroughly combined (I use my hands to do this). Let the mixture sit for a couple of minutes to allow the flours to fully absorb the liquid. Add the beaten egg and mix again with your hands until everything is thoroughly combined.

5 Pour the crust mixture into the middle of the tart pan. Using a small offset spatula or your hands, spread the mixture until it covers the base and the sides of the pan evenly. Bake until the edges begin to crisp, 12 to 15 minutes. Remove from the oven and turn down the heat to 375°F (190°C).

6 Now, make the preserves. Mix the gelatin and lemon juice in a small bowl. Set aside.

7 Place the 1 tablespoon (15 ml) coconut oil and 1 cup (150 g) of the blueberries in a medium saucepan over medium heat. Cook, stirring often, until the blueberries begin to burst, about 5 minutes. Turn the heat to low and add the lemon-gelatin mixture, whisking until the gelatin is completely dissolved, about 1 minute.

8 Remove from the heat and stir in the honey or syrup, salt, and the remaining 2 cups (300 g) blueberries.

9 Spread the blueberry preserves over the top of the tart crust. Layer the caramelized onions over the preserves. Top with as much goat cheese as you'd like. Bake the tart until the cheese begins to soften, 8 to 10 minutes. Garnish with the basil before serving.

PREP TIME:
10 minutes

COOK TIME:
30 minutes

YIELD:
6 servings

patatas bravas

3 pounds (1.4 kg) Yukon
  gold or red potatoes, cut
  into 1-inch (2.5 cm) cubes
¼ cup (60 ml) avocado oil
Kosher salt, to taste
Black pepper, to taste
Chopped fresh parsley, for
  garnish
½ cup (115 g) Tomato-Garlic
  Aioli (page 182)

This traditional Spanish tapa is basically seasoned fried
potatoes, often served with a creamy-spicy sauce. I've created
this paleo version, paired with my Tomato-Garlic Aioli, and
it's absolutely fantastic. It's reminiscent of true comfort food
but it won't leave you feeling like you need to take a nap.

1 Preheat the oven to 425°F (220°C) and adjust the oven rack to the
   middle position. Line two baking sheets with parchment paper.

2 In a large bowl, toss the potato cubes with the oil, using your hands
   or a spoon until they are evenly coated. Season with salt and pepper.

3 Spread the potatoes onto both parchment-lined baking sheets. Make
   sure they have some room and are in an even and flat layer on each sheet.

4 Roast until the potatoes begin to turn golden brown, 25 to 30 minutes.
   Turn the oven to a low broil for 4 minutes, keeping a close eye to make
   sure the potatoes do not burn. Rotate the baking sheets 180 degrees
   halfway through.

5 Remove the potatoes from the oven and transfer to a serving platter to
   slightly cool. Sprinkle with the parsley and serve the aioli on the side.

NOTE:

If you can't fit two baking
sheets side by side in
your oven, adjust the
racks to the upper and
lower thirds, and switch
the sheets halfway
through baking. To broil,
they will have to be done
one at a time.

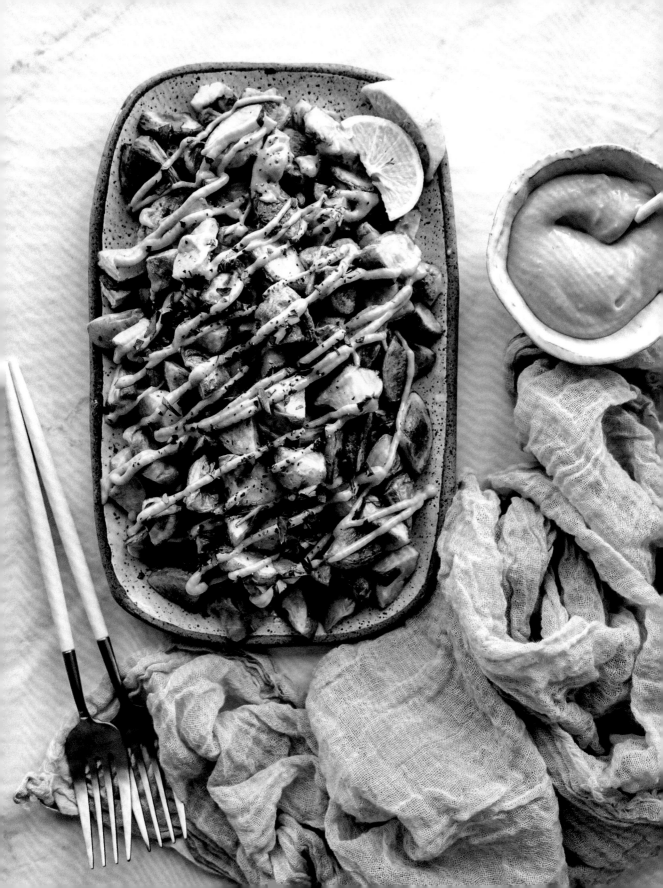

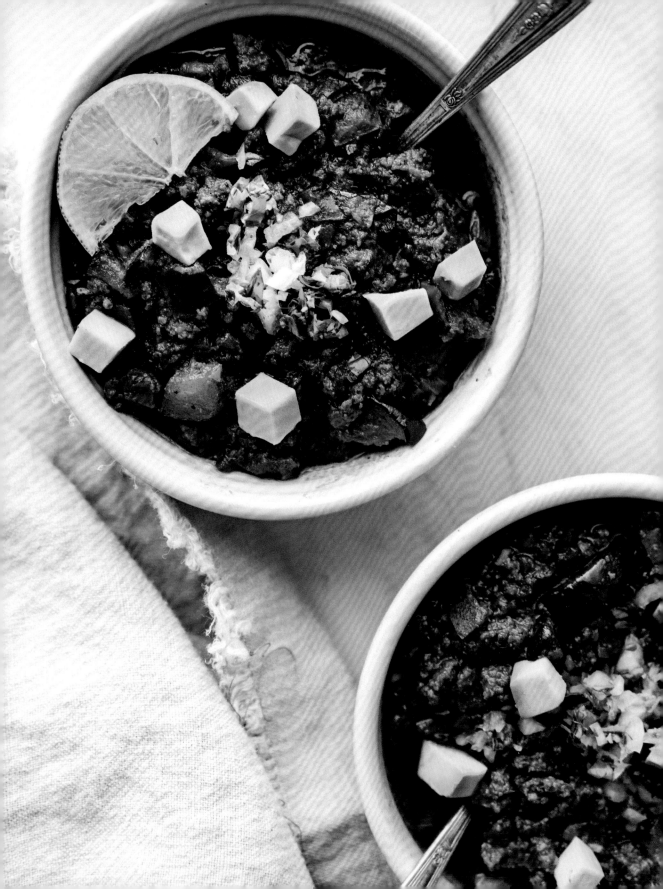

one-pan/ one-pot meals

THERE IS SOMETHING SO DANG MAGICAL ABOUT making a meal all in one cooking vessel, isn't there? I'm always impressed when something so beautiful and delicious can be the product of such a small mess with very little cleanup. It makes me immediately excited when thinking about my next meal, as I'm not exhausted from the amount of time I spent in the kitchen. That's a win in my book.

I've included a variety of different cooking methods in this chapter, from oven to stove top to Instant Pot. For those recipes that call for an Instant Pot, you can use a slow cooker instead, or you can cook it on the stove—it just might take a little longer. I'm covering all my bases here.

You'll find all kinds of one-pan goodness in this chapter, from dishes like One-Pan Shrimp Fajitas and Drunken Zucchini Noodles to Steak & Veggie Stir-Fry and Clean Paleo Chicken Curry. (Not coincidently, these are some of my favorites.) I can't wait for you to dive in!

◀ Clean Paleo Chili, page 92

PREP TIME:
15 minutes

COOK TIME:
15 minutes

YIELD:
6 servings

chicken mole lettuce wraps

2 tablespoons (30 ml) avocado oil

1 yellow onion, diced

8 cloves garlic, minced

1 can (14.5 ounces [408 g]) fire-roasted crushed tomatoes

Handful of raw cashews

¼ cup (40 g) pepitas, plus more, toasted, for topping

3 tablespoons (45 ml) chicken bone broth or chicken broth

3 tablespoons (21 g) unsweetened raisins

2½ tablespoons (12.5 g) cacao powder

2 tablespoons (15 g) ancho chile powder

1 tablespoon (16 g) tomato paste

1 tablespoon (15 ml) apple cider vinegar

1 teaspoon (2.5 g) paprika

1 teaspoon (6 g) kosher salt, plus more to taste

¼ teaspoon ground cumin

⅛ teaspoon coriander powder

⅛ teaspoon anise powder

Pinch of dried oregano

Pinch of ground cloves

Black pepper, to taste

2 pounds (900 g) boneless, skinless chicken thighs

1 cinnamon stick

Butter lettuce leaves, for serving

Chopped fresh parsley, for topping

Coconut yogurt, for topping

Sliced red onion, for topping

While a traditional mole sauce can take hours to prepare, you don't need to spend all day over the stove to make this super flavorful and pronounced sauce at home. It's made with pepitas, cashews, raisins, and cacao powder, but don't let the long list of ingredients intimidate you—simply have it ready to go before you begin cooking. You are going to be so impressed with yourself after making this chicken and sauce that's so warm, nourishing, bright, and sassy. Wrap it in some butter lettuce and garnish with the recommended toppings. It's a guaranteed win!

1 Set the Instant Pot to the Sauté function and add the oil. Once it is hot, add the onion and garlic. Sauté until the onion is soft and the garlic is quite fragrant, 3 to 4 minutes. Press Cancel.

2 Transfer the onion mixture to the pitcher of a high-speed blender and add the tomatoes, cashews, pepitas, broth, raisins, cacao, ancho chile, tomato paste, vinegar, paprika, salt, cumin, coriander, anise, oregano, cloves, and a few grinds of black pepper. Blend on medium-high speed until creamy throughout.

3 Add the chicken to the Instant Pot. Pour the mole mixture all over the chicken and add the cinnamon stick. Set the Instant Pot to pressure Cook (Manual) on High, and set the time to 15 minutes.

4 Once it's done, let the pressure release naturally for 10 minutes. Manually let the pressure out, covering the steam with a kitchen towel. Using two forks, shred and break apart the chicken and mix well into the sauce. Remove the cinnamon stick and discard.

5 Be sure to taste and adjust the seasoning levels. You will likely need to add more salt to your taste preferences.

6 Add the chicken mole to butter lettuce leaves and garnish with your desired toppings. Serve warm.

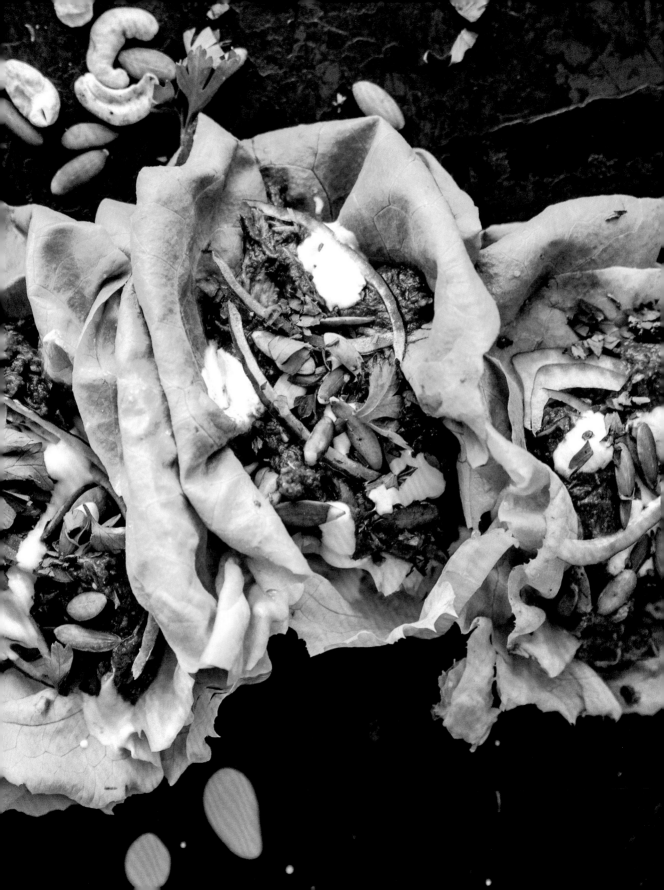

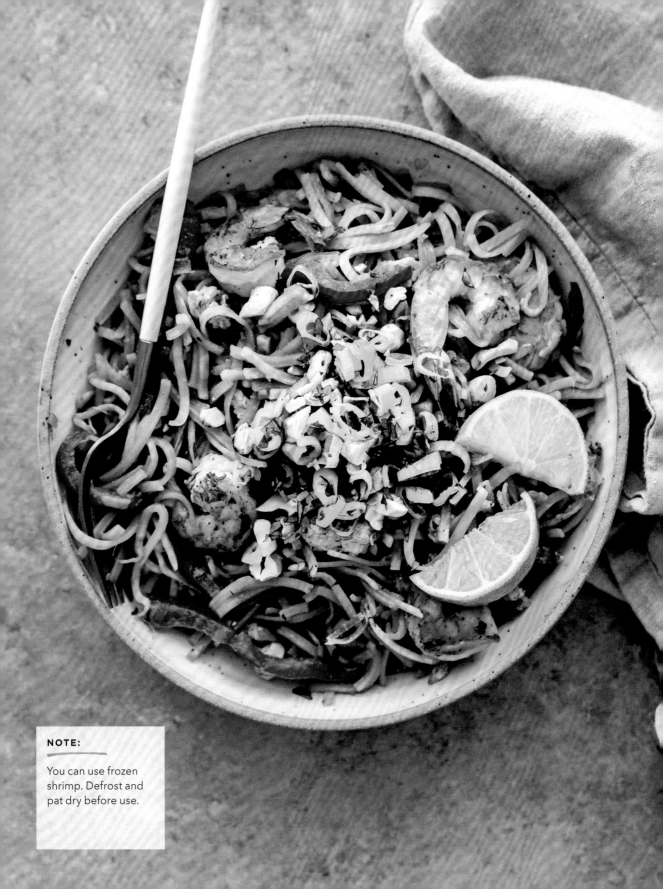

NOTE:

You can use frozen
shrimp. Defrost and
pat dry before use.

PREP TIME:
15 minutes

COOK TIME:
20 minutes

YIELD:
4 to 6 servings

SWEETENER / GRAIN

rice noodle shrimp pad thai

8 ounces (225 g) rice noodles

SAUCE
¼ cup (50 g) coconut sugar
3 tablespoons (45 ml)
    fish sauce
3 tablespoons (45 ml)
    coconut aminos
2 tablespoons (30 ml)
    rice vinegar
2 tablespoon (30 g)
    cashew butter
1 tablespoon (15 ml)
    hot sauce

PAD THAI
4 tablespoons (60 ml)
    avocado oil, divided
1 pound (450 g) large shrimp,
    peeled, deveined, and
    patted dry (see Note)
2 large eggs
1 teaspoon (5 ml) filtered
    water
2 small red bell peppers,
    julienned
6 cloves garlic, minced
1½ cups (150 g) tightly
    packed bean sprouts
5 scallions, sliced (reserve
    some for garnish)
½ cup (75 g) dry-roasted
    cashews, chopped
    (reserve some for garnish)
2 limes, cut into wedges

A rice noodle shrimp pad Thai recipe with all of the bold flavors and none of the filler ingredients? Sign me up! The sauce for this dish is absolutely delectable and is made from a short list of ingredients. Use your favorite protein if shrimp aren't your thing, but it's the dry-roasted cashews and scallions that really round out the flavors.

1   Prepare the rice noodles according to package directions. Drain.

2   To make the sauce, in a small bowl, whisk together the coconut sugar, fish sauce, coconut aminos, vinegar, cashew butter, and hot sauce until well combined. If your cashew butter isn't creamy, you may see some chunks, and that is fine.

3   To make the pad thai, heat a large skillet over medium heat and add 2 tablespoons (30 ml) of the oil. When hot (about 2 minutes), add the shrimp in a single layer. Be sure not to overcrowd. Cook until opaque and the tails have curled, 2 to 3 minutes per side, and transfer to a plate or bowl.

4   In a small bowl, whisk together the eggs and water. Return the skillet to medium heat and add another 1 tablespoon (15 ml) oil. Pour in the eggs and cook undisturbed until no longer runny, about 2 minutes. Transfer the egg to a plate and roughly break apart with a fork.

5   Add the remaining 1 tablespoon (15 ml) oil to the skillet and return to medium heat. Add the peppers and garlic and cook until slightly softened, stirring occasionally, 4 minutes.

6   Add the prepared noodles, bean sprouts, scallions (reserving a handful), and cashews (reserving a handful). Cook until the veggies are soft and the flavors have melded together, 3 to 4 minutes. Add the sauce and cook for another 5 minutes, stirring often. Add the shrimp and eggs back to the pan and stir occasionally for 2 more minutes to heat.

7   Top with more cashews, scallions, and a squeeze of lime before serving.

PREP TIME:
30 minutes
COOK TIME:
25 minutes
YIELD:
4 servings

steak & veggie stir-fry

2 small Japanese eggplants, cut into ½-inch (1 cm) half-moons (about 3 cups [450 g])

About 2 tablespoons (36 g) plus 2 teaspoons (12 g) kosher salt, divided

1½ pounds (680 g) skirt steak, thinly sliced across the grain

2 teaspoons (10 ml) plus 4 tablespoons (60 ml) coconut oil, divided

1 tablespoon (8 g) arrowroot flour

½ teaspoon black pepper

1 small yellow onion, sliced

2 cups (300 g) broccoli florets

3 medium carrots, sliced ¼ inch (6 mm) thick

1 red bell pepper, julienned

¾ cup (110 g) sugar snap peas, trimmed

1 batch Asian Marinade/ Stir-Fry Sauce (page 175)

⅓ cup (50 g) thinly sliced scallions, for garnish

White sesame seeds, for garnish

This stir-fry is full of so much flavor, you'll be shocked it comes together so easily. You're going to want everything ready—including the stir-fry sauce—before you put the pan on the heat. This dish is loaded with umami from the stir-fry sauce, and the crust you'll get on the skirt steak is seriously irresistible. This works great if you're meal prepping, but it would also be perfect for a dinner with friends.

1   Place the eggplant in a colander and set it in the sink. Add 2 tablespoons (36 g) of the salt and mix well with your hands. Let it sit and release excess water for 20 minutes. Rinse well with cold water and pat very dry with a towel. Set aside.

2   Meanwhile, in a medium bowl, combine the steak, 2 teaspoons (10 ml) of the oil, arrowroot, 1½ teaspoons (9 g) salt, and black pepper. Toss to evenly coat and set aside for 5 minutes.

3   Heat a large, high-sided sauté pan over high heat for 1 minute and add 2 tablespoons (30 ml) oil. Heat for 1 minute. Add the steak in two batches, making sure it is spread out evenly in a single layer. Sear for about 2 minutes and flip over. Cook for another 30 seconds to 1 minute, just until browned, and transfer to a plate or bowl.

4   Wipe out the pan with a paper towel and add 1 tablespoon (15 ml) oil. Turn the heat to medium-high. Add the onion and cook until soft, stirring occasionally, 4 to 5 minutes.

5   Add the remaining 1 tablespoon (15 ml) oil along with the eggplant, broccoli, and remaining ½ teaspoon salt. Cook until crisp-tender, 5 to 6 minutes. Add the carrots, bell pepper, and snap peas. Cook for 5 to 7 minutes, stirring occasionally, until the veggies have cooked through and are relatively fork tender. Stir in the steak.

6   Add the stir-fry sauce and reduce the heat to medium. Cook until the sauce is evenly dispersed and has reduced slightly, 3 to 5 minutes. Serve right away, garnished with the scallions and sesame seeds.

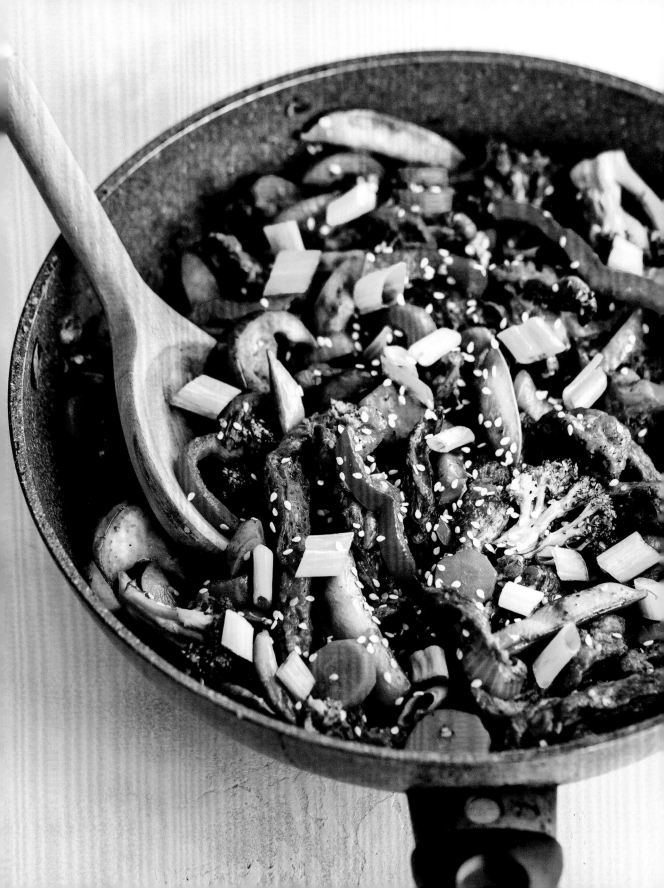

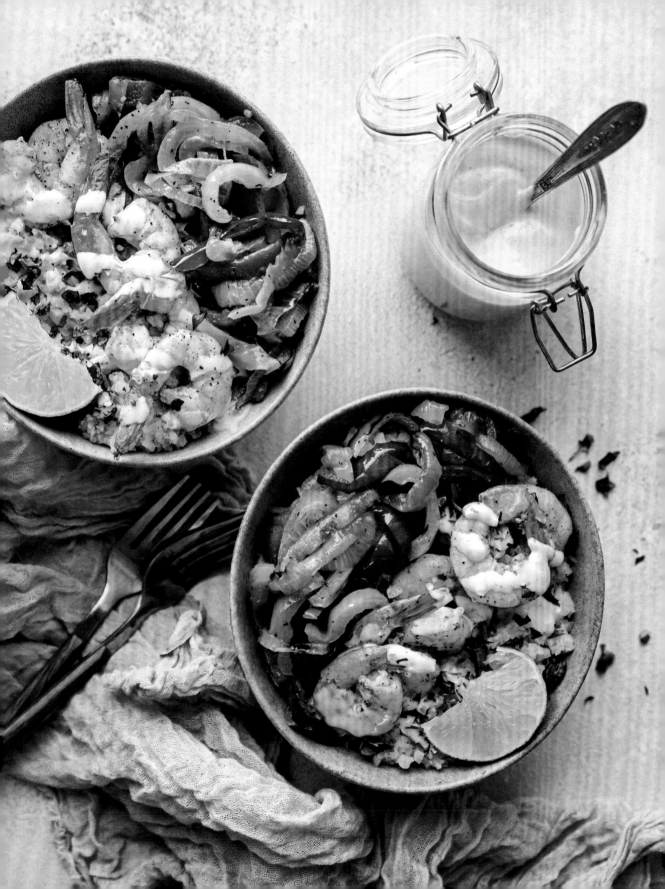

PREP TIME:
15 minutes

COOK TIME:
25 minutes

YIELD:
4 servings

one-pan shrimp fajitas

SHRIMP

3 tablespoons (45 ml) avocado oil
1 lime, juiced
6 cloves garlic, minced
1 teaspoon (6 g) kosher salt
½ teaspoon black pepper
½ teaspoon paprika
½ teaspoon chili powder
½ teaspoon ground cinnamon
Pinch of crushed red pepper flakes
1½ pounds (680 g) extra-large shrimp, peeled, deveined, and tails removed

PEPPERS & ONIONS

3 bell peppers (1 each red, yellow, green), sliced
1 yellow onion, sliced
1½ tablespoons (22 ml) avocado oil
Kosher salt, to taste
Black pepper, to taste

COCONUT CAULIFLOWER RICE

3 cups (450 g) cauliflower rice
¼ cup (60 ml) full-fat canned coconut milk
2 tablespoons (30 ml) fresh lime juice
1 tablespoon (15 ml) avocado oil
¼ teaspoon kosher salt
⅓ cup (5 g) finely chopped cilantro

These shrimp fajitas come together almost magically. The coconut cauliflower rice pairs perfectly with the sizzling shrimp and peppers. There's very little cleanup and lots of flavor—the best one-pan dish!

1 Preheat the oven to 450°F (230°C) and adjust the oven rack to the middle position. Line a baking sheet with parchment paper.

2 To make the shrimp, in a medium bowl, whisk together the oil, lime juice, garlic, salt, black pepper, paprika, chili powder, cinnamon, and red pepper flakes. Add the shrimp and toss thoroughly to completely coat the shrimp. Set aside.

3 To make the peppers and onions, spread the bell peppers and onion in an even layer on the prepared baking sheet. Add the oil and toss thoroughly to coat everything. Sprinkle with salt and black pepper. Roast until soft throughout, 12 to 15 minutes.

4 Meanwhile, prepare the rice. In a small bowl, combine the cauliflower, coconut milk, lime juice, oil, and salt. Taste for additional seasoning.

5 Remove the peppers and onions from the oven and move them to one third of the baking sheet. Add the cauliflower rice to the opposite side (one third of the sheet).

6 Pour the shrimp and marinade into the center of the baking sheet. Return the pan to the oven and roast until the shrimp have cooked through and look opaque, another 10 to 12 minutes. Remove from the oven and stir the cilantro into the rice. Serve right away.

PREP TIME:
20 minutes
COOK TIME:
30 minutes
YIELD:
6 to 8 servings

clean paleo chicken curry

1½ tablespoons (22 ml) ghee or avocado oil, divided
1½ pounds (680 g) boneless, skinless chicken thighs, patted dry and cut into 1-inch (2.5 cm) cubes
Kosher salt, to taste
Black pepper, to taste
¼ cup (60 ml) chicken bone broth or low-sodium chicken broth
1 small yellow onion, diced
¼ cup (60 g) green curry paste
3 cans (13.5 ounces [395 ml]) full-fat coconut milk
1 head cauliflower, cut into small florets
2 cups (300 g) trimmed green beans
2 cups (300 g) diced butternut squash
2 teaspoons (6 g) garlic powder
2 teaspoons (4 g) curry powder
1 teaspoon (1.2 g) crushed red pepper flakes
¾ teaspoon ground ginger
2 teaspoons (4.4 g) turmeric powder
Fresh chopped cilantro, for serving

This flavor-forward, easy chicken curry is made with all kinds of spices and nutrient-dense veggies. Try it once and you'll find yourself making this pretty curry time and time again. Serve it with cauliflower rice, rice, or naan bread.

1   Heat a high-sided sauté pan with 1 tablespoon (15 ml) of the ghee or oil over medium-high heat. While it is heating up, sprinkle the chicken with salt and black pepper.

2   Panfry the chicken until lightly brown on all sides, 4 to 5 minutes (it doesn't have to cook through). Using a slotted spoon, transfer the pieces to a bowl and set aside. Discard the excess fat and juice from the pan.

3   Add the broth and onion to the pan and cook until translucent, 4 to 5 minutes.

4   Add the remaining ½ tablespoon (7.5 ml) oil to the pan to heat. Add the chicken and the curry paste. Stir until well combined and pour in the coconut milk. Let it just come to a boil and turn down the heat to medium-low.

5   Add the cauliflower, green beans, squash, garlic powder, curry powder, red pepper flakes, and ginger. Stir to combine and simmer until the vegetables are fork tender, about 12 minutes. Stir in turmeric.

6   Add salt and black pepper, to taste.

7   Let the curry simmer until all of the veggies are very tender and the sauce has thickened up a bit, 15 to 20 minutes. Mix in or garnish with fresh cilantro before serving.

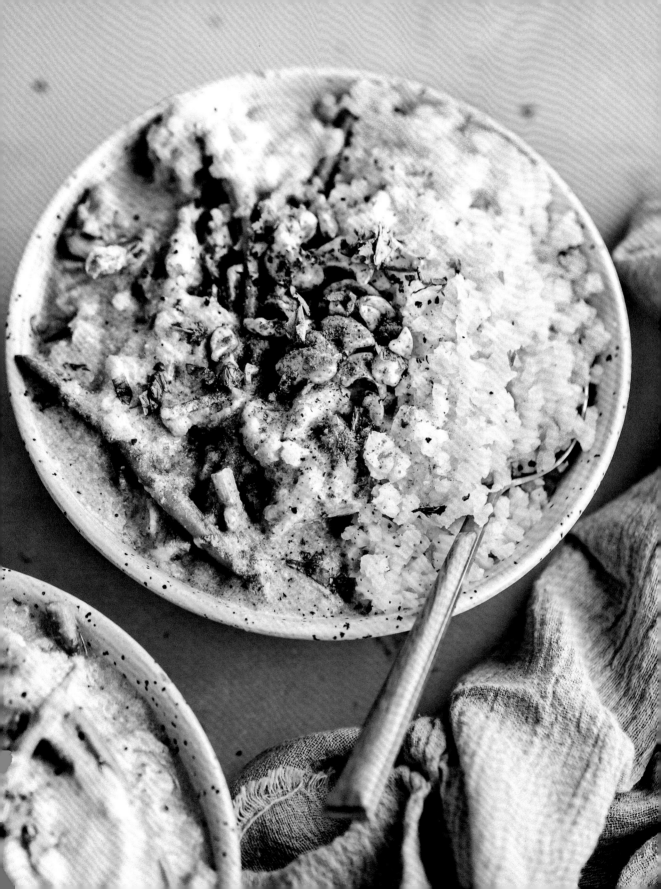

PREP TIME:
15 minutes

COOK TIME:
20 minutes

YIELD:
4 servings

asian salmon with potatoes & broccoli

- 3 tablespoons (45 ml) toasted sesame oil
- 1 tablespoon plus ¼ cup (75 ml) coconut aminos, divided
- 1 teaspoon (3 g) garlic powder
- ¾ teaspoon kosher salt, divided, plus more to taste
- 2 pounds (900 g) Yukon gold potatoes, cut into 1½-inch (4 cm) chunks
- 2 tablespoons (30 ml) avocado oil
- 1 tablespoon (15 ml) rice vinegar
- ½ pound (600 g) broccoli florets (about 4 cups)
- 3 tablespoons (45 ml) Clean Paleo Mayo (page 176)
- 1 pound (450 g) salmon, cut into 4 even portions
- Black pepper, to taste
- 2 scallions, thinly sliced on the diagonal, for garnish

One-pan meals may be all the rage, but this dish has so much flavor, you're going to want it for lunch *and* dinner. Double up and use two sheet pans if you can. Not only is this salmon recipe an awesome one-dish dinner, but it's also perfect for meal prep, as it still tastes wonderful when reheated as leftovers.

1 Preheat the oven to 425°F (220°C) and adjust the oven rack to the middle position. Coat a large rimmed baking sheet with oil.

2 In a large bowl, mix together the sesame oil, 1 tablespoon (15 ml) of the coconut aminos, garlic powder, and ½ teaspoon of the salt. Add the potatoes and mix thoroughly with your hands so everything is evenly coated. Transfer in a single layer to the prepared baking sheet. Roast for 20 minutes.

3 Meanwhile, in the same bowl, mix together the remaining ¼ cup (60 ml) coconut aminos, avocado oil, vinegar, and remaining ¼ teaspoon salt. Transfer 2 tablespoons (30 ml) of this marinade to a small bowl. Add the broccoli to the bowl with the remaining marinade and toss to combine.

4 Remove the potatoes from the oven, flip the potatoes over, and make room for the broccoli and salmon. Add the broccoli to the baking sheet.

5 For the salmon, mix together the reserved marinade with the mayo until smooth throughout. Set the salmon on the baking sheet and sprinkle with salt and pepper. Using a brush, coat the salmon evenly with the mayo-marinade mixture.

6 Return the baking sheet to the oven and cook until the salmon flakes easily with a fork, 12 to 15 minutes. Garnish with the scallions before serving.

PREP TIME:
15 minutes
COOK TIME:
20 minutes
YIELD:
6 to 8 servings

beef bolognese

- 8 medium zucchini (see Note)
- 2 tablespoons (36 g) kosher salt, plus more to taste
- 6 strips bacon, finely diced
- 4 carrots, diced
- 3 ribs celery, diced
- 1 yellow onion, diced
- 8 cloves garlic, minced
- 2 pounds (900 g) grass-fed 90/10 or 92/8 ground beef
- 2 cans (6 ounces [169 g]) tomato paste
- 1 cup (240 ml) full-fat canned coconut milk
- 1 cup (240 ml) chicken bone broth or low-sodium chicken broth
- 2 teaspoons (6 g) garlic powder
- Black pepper, to taste

NOTE:

If you don't have a spiralizer, buy about 2½ pounds (1125 g) precut zoodles.

This wonderful Clean Paleo beef Bolognese is going to blow your mind. It can all be prepared in one pan, comes together oh so quickly, and has so much flavor, you'd think it had been cooking for days. Be sure to double the batch if you want to save on meal prep. It freezes extremely well and tastes delicious reheated!

1 Spiralize the zucchini first, as thick or as thin as you'd like. Add the zucchini to a large colander in the sink. Add the salt and massage it into the zucchini. Let it sit for about 20 minutes, as this process will release a lot of moisture. Rinse the zucchini well with cold water and let it drain for another 10 to 15 minutes. Pat it as dry as you can with a kitchen towel and set aside.

2 Meanwhile, cook the bacon in a large pot over medium-high heat until crunchy, stirring often, about 4 minutes. Transfer the bacon to a paper towel–lined plate.

3 Lower the heat to medium. Add the carrots, celery, and onion to the pot and cook, stirring occasionally, until the onion appears translucent, about 5 minutes. Add the garlic and cook for another minute or so, until fragrant.

4 Add the beef and cook, breaking up the pieces, until brown, about 5 minutes. Stir in the tomato paste, coconut milk, broth, and reserved bacon. Bring to a simmer and cook until it thickens, 7 to 10 minutes.

5 Stir in the garlic powder, along with salt and black pepper, to taste.

6 Stir in the zucchini noodles and let everything cook together for 4 to 5 minutes. Serve warm.

PREP TIME:
10 minutes
COOK TIME:
30 minutes
YIELD:
4 servings

clean paleo chili

2 tablespoons (30 ml) avocado oil

2 bell peppers (any color), cut into 1-inch (2.5 cm) chunks

1 medium zucchini, cut into 1-inch (2.5 cm) chunks (about 2 cups [300 g])

1 white onion, diced

1½ tablespoons (10.7 g) chili powder

1½ teaspoons (3.7 g) ground cumin

1½ teaspoons (2.7 g) dried oregano

1 teaspoon (2.4 g) onion powder

1 teaspoon (6 g) garlic powder

1 teaspoon (2.3 g) ground cinnamon

1 teaspoon (6 g) kosher salt, plus more to taste

6 cloves garlic, minced

1 pound (450 g) grass-fed 85/15 or 90/10 ground beef (see Notes)

1 can (14.5 ounces [408 g]) fire-roasted diced tomatoes

1 cup (240 ml) tomato sauce

1 can (4 ounces [113 g]) diced green chiles

¼ cup (60 ml) cold brew coffee (see Notes)

¾ cup (180 ml) chicken or beef bone broth (see Notes)

Black pepper, to taste

This Clean Paleo chili has some special ingredients to bring it above and beyond other chilis you've tried. I mean, cold brew coffee and cinnamon in chili? Heck, yes! The bold and bright flavors will really wow you. You can make it quickly in an Instant Pot or low and slow on the stove top. Either way, serve with fresh chopped herbs, diced avocado, and more onions!

INSTANT POT

1 Turn on the Instant Pot and press the Sauté function. Add the oil to the pot and let it heat up for 2 minutes.

2 Add the bell peppers, zucchini, onion, chili powder, cumin, oregano, onion powder, garlic powder, cinnamon, and salt. Sauté until the veggies are fragrant and soft throughout, stirring occasionally, 7 to 9 minutes. Add the garlic and sauté for 1 additional minute.

3 Add the ground beef and break it up with a wooden utensil, stirring frequently, until browned throughout, 3 to 4 minutes.

4 Add the tomatoes, tomato sauce, green chiles (with their juice), coffee, and broth and stir. Press Keep Warm/Cancel. Cover and set to Sealing. Press Manual and cook for 20 minutes on High.

5 When finished, release the pressure naturally for 15 minutes. Cautiously change to Venting to manually release the pressure. When released, remove the lid, taste for additional salt and black pepper, and serve.

STOVE TOP

1 Heat the oil in a stockpot or Dutch oven over medium heat.

2 Once hot, follow step 2 of Instant Pot instructions.

3 Add the ground beef and cook until the meat turns slightly brown, 3 to 4 minutes. Drain out the excess fat/liquid, if you'd like.

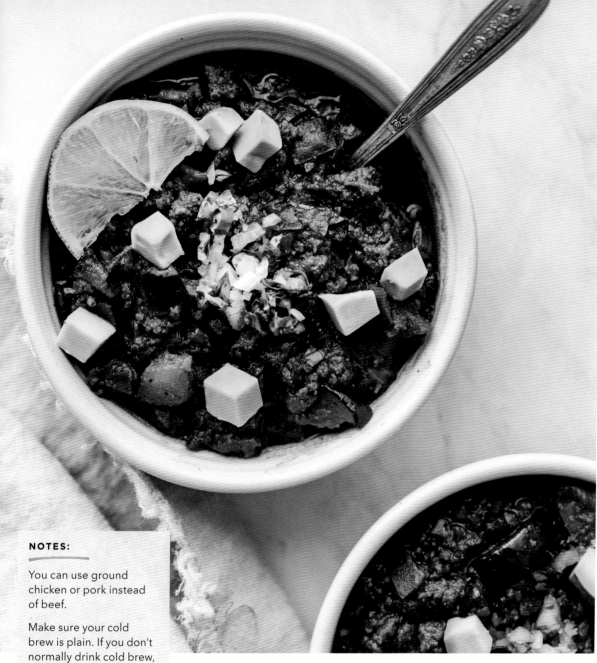

NOTES:

You can use ground chicken or pork instead of beef.

Make sure your cold brew is plain. If you don't normally drink cold brew, make a pot of very strong coffee, two to three times the strength you'd normally brew.

You can use chicken or beef stock instead of bone broth.

4 Add the tomatoes, tomato sauce, green chiles, coffee, and broth. Bring to a boil, then lower the heat and simmer, stirring occasionally, for 2 hours.

5 Taste for additional salt and black pepper, and serve.

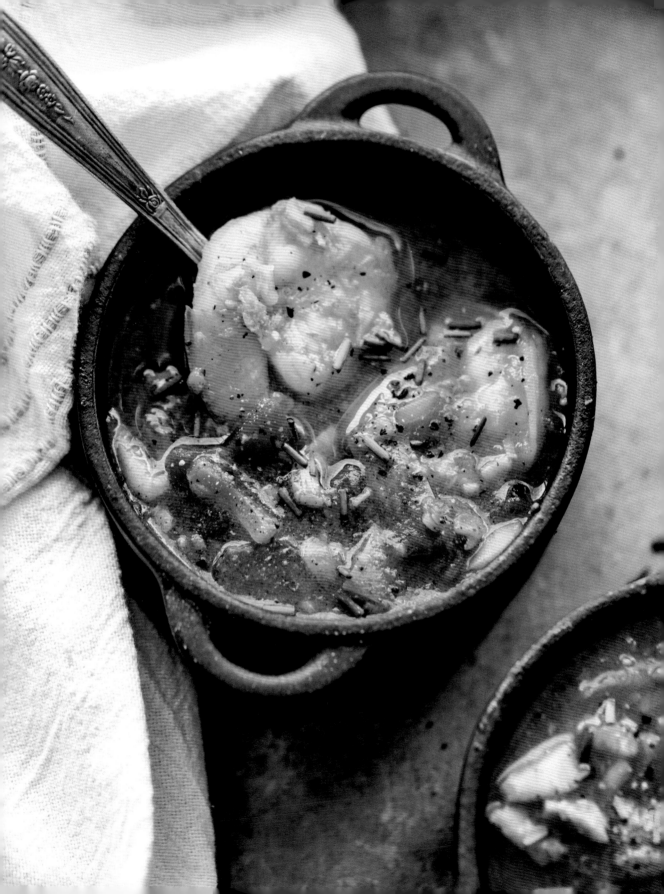

PREP TIME:
10 minutes
COOK TIME:
25 minutes
YIELD:
8 to 10 servings

instant pot gumbo

1½ pounds (680 g) wild-caught cod, patted dry and cut into 2-inch (5 cm) chunks

Kosher salt, to taste

Black pepper, to taste

3 tablespoons (10.8 g) Cajun or Creole seasoning, divided

3 tablespoons (45 ml) ghee or avocado oil

4 ribs celery, diced

2 yellow onions, diced

2 green bell peppers, diced

1 can (28 ounces [793 g]) diced tomatoes

1½ cups (350 ml) chicken broth

¼ cup (65 g) tomato paste

3 bay leaves

1½ pounds (680 g) medium or large shrimp, peeled and deveined

Chopped chives or scallion greens, for serving

My take on gumbo doesn't include a traditional roux, but it sure does come bursting with flavor from traditional ingredients like white fish, bell peppers, and shrimp! It's the perfect one-pot meal to add into your rotation that's both paleo and low carb. Serve it with cauliflower rice or regular rice, and it tastes even more fabulous the next day—even cold!

1 Sprinkle the cod with salt and black pepper, making sure the pieces are as evenly coated as possible. Sprinkle half the Cajun seasoning evenly onto the fish.

2 Add the ghee to the Instant Pot and press Sauté. When it reads Hot, add the fish. Sauté until it looks cooked on all sides, about 4 minutes. Use a slotted spoon to transfer the fish to a large plate.

3 Add the celery, onions, bell peppers, and the remaining Cajun seasoning to the pot and sauté until fragrant, 2 minutes. Press Keep Warm/Cancel.

4 Add the fish, tomatoes, broth, tomato paste, and bay leaves and give it a nice stir. Put the lid back on the pot and set it to Sealing. Press Manual and set the time for 5 minutes. (The Instant Pot will slowly build up to a high-pressure point and once it reaches that point, the gumbo will cook for 5 minutes.)

5 Once it's finished cooking, press the Keep Warm/Cancel button. Cautiously change the Sealing valve over to Venting, which will manually release all the pressure.

6 Once the pressure has been released (this will take a couple of minutes), remove the lid and change the setting to Sauté again. Add the shrimp and cook until the shrimp become opaque and the tails curl, 3 to 4 minutes. Remove the bay leaves and add more salt and black pepper, to taste. Serve topped with chives or scallion greens.

PREP TIME:
15 minutes
COOK TIME:
30 minutes
YIELD:
6 to 8 servings

drunken zucchini noodles

NOODLES

8 medium zucchini (see Notes, page 98)

2 tablespoons (36 g) plus ½ teaspoon kosher salt, divided

2 pounds (900 g) boneless, skinless chicken thighs, patted dry and cut into 1½-inch (4 cm) chunks

½ teaspoon black pepper, plus more to taste

1½ tablespoons (12 g) arrowroot flour

3 tablespoons (45 ml) ghee or coconut oil, divided

3 carrots, sliced

2 cups (300 g) broccoli florets

1 yellow onion, diced

3 red bell peppers, sliced

1 cup (150 g) snow peas, trimmed

2 teaspoons (6 g) minced garlic

1 cup (24 g) Thai basil, chopped, plus more for garnish

3 Thai chiles, minced, plus more for garnish

(continued)

I've got a better-for-you rendition of a traditional drunken noodles recipe. It's made with zucchini noodles (instead of rice noodles), plenty of fabulous vegetables, and juicy chicken. The sauce is absolutely to die for and is bursting with umami. The zing, robust flavors, and overall goodness coming from this dish are going to knock your socks off, and I can't wait for you to wow yourself when you make it.

1   To make the noodles, spiralize the zucchini as thick or as thin as you'd like. Add the spiralized zucchini to a large colander in the sink. Add 2 tablespoons (36 g) of the salt and massage it into the zucchini. Let it sit for about 20 minutes, as this process will release a lot of moisture. Rinse the zucchini well with cold water and let it drain for another 10 to 15 minutes. Pat it as dry as you can with a kitchen towel and set aside.

2   Meanwhile, sprinkle the chicken with the remaining ½ teaspoon salt and black pepper and coat with the arrowroot flour. Add half the oil to a large skillet over medium-high heat, tilting it to coat the entire surface. Once hot, a couple of minutes, add the chicken. Cook until cooked through, (go ahead and grab a piece and cut it in half to double-check!), 7 to 10 minutes. Using a slotted spoon, transfer the chicken to a large bowl.

3   Add the remaining oil to the skillet and toss in the carrots, broccoli, and onion. Cook over medium-high heat, stirring occasionally, until the carrots are soft when pierced with a fork, about 7 minutes. Add the bell peppers and snow peas. Cook until they are a little bit soft, 3 to 5 minutes. Add the garlic and stir until fragrant, 30 seconds. Add the basil and chiles. Reduce the heat to medium-low and cook for 2 to 3 minutes, stirring frequently.

(continued)

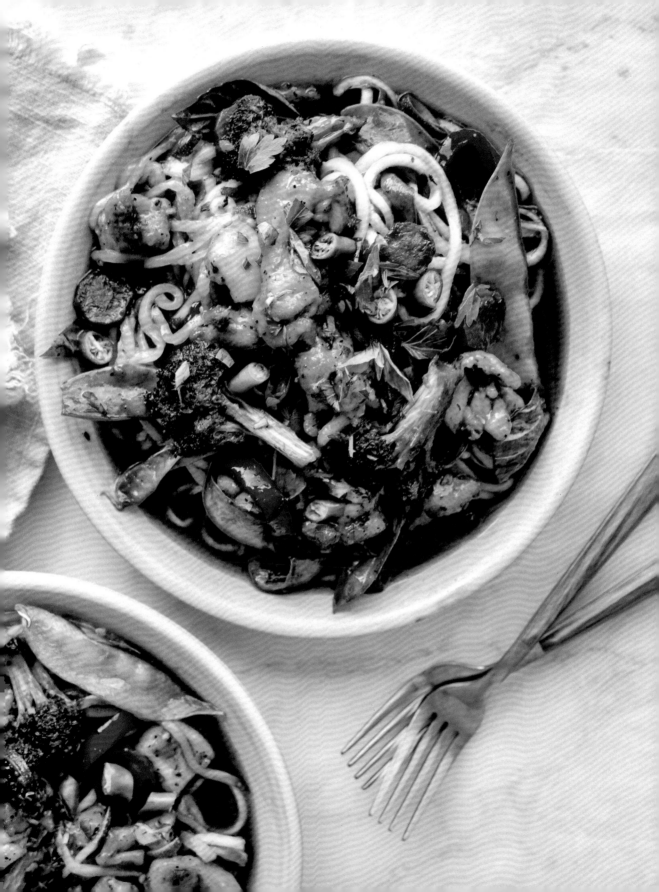

SAUCE

1 cup (240 ml) coconut aminos

¼ cup (60 g) chili garlic paste (see Notes)

¼ cup (60 ml) fish sauce

1 heaping teaspoon (2 g) minced fresh ginger

1 teaspoon (1.2 g) crushed red pepper flakes

1 lime, juiced, plus lime wedges for garnish

½ lime, zested

2 teaspoons (16 g) arrowroot flour

1½ teaspoons (7.5 ml) filtered water

NOTES:

If you don't have a spiralizer, buy about 2½ pounds (1.1 kg) precut zoodles.

Look for a chili garlic paste without any MSG, sugar, or preservatives.

4 As the stir-fry is cooking, prepare the sauce. In a medium bowl, whisk together the coconut aminos, chili garlic paste, fish sauce, ginger, red pepper flakes, lime juice, and lime zest.

5 Once the vegetables are cooked, add the cooked chicken back to the skillet and stir everything together.

6 Stir in the sauce and turn the heat to medium. Once the mixture begins to simmer, turn the heat to medium-low and cook for 5 minutes. Add the spiralized zucchini and cook until the noodles have reached your desired level of doneness, about 5 minutes.

7 In a small bowl, mix the arrowroot flour with water until smooth. Slowly drizzle into the noodles, stirring frequently. You may add a little bit more if you'd like the sauce even thicker.

8 Serve with fresh squeezed lime, Thai chiles, and Thai basil as garnish.

PREP TIME:
15 minutes

COOK TIME:
25 minutes

YIELD:
4 servings

skillet chicken with brussels sprouts & apples

3 tablespoons (45 ml) avocado oil, divided

1½ pounds (680 g) boneless, skinless chicken thighs

1 tablespoon (2.7 g) fresh thyme, chopped

Kosher salt, to taste

Black pepper, to taste

12 ounces (453 g) Brussels sprouts, shredded

1 apple, thinly sliced

½ small red onion, diced

4 cloves garlic, minced

3 tablespoons (45 ml) coconut aminos

2 tablespoons (30 ml) rice vinegar

1 tablespoon (15 ml) sesame oil

½ cup (75 g) pecans, chopped and toasted (see Note)

I love this skillet chicken so much because the Brussels sprouts, apples, and pecans give me serious Thanksgiving and Christmas vibes. My husband's family is Vietnamese, and it's no secret that I like to make Asian-influenced dishes. I've mashed up these holiday vibes and family influences in one dish, and our daughter, Sophie, loses her mind over these flavors. This simple skillet is really just a fabulous, warm, and comforting dish to enjoy year-round. May it become full of nostalgia for you as well.

1 Heat a large skillet over medium-high heat. Add half the avocado oil and heat for 1 minute. Meanwhile, sprinkle the chicken with the thyme and a big pinch of salt and pepper.

2 Add the chicken to the skillet in a single layer. You may need to work in two batches depending on the size of your skillet. Cook until the chicken reaches an internal temperature of 165°F (74°C), 4 to 5 minutes per side. Transfer to a plate.

3 Add the remaining avocado oil to the skillet, along with the Brussels sprouts, apple, and onion. Cook until the Brussels sprouts have wilted and the onion is soft, about 5 minutes. Add the garlic and cook, stirring frequently, for 1 minute.

4 Stir in the coconut aminos, vinegar, and sesame oil. Cook until quite fragrant, 2 to 3 minutes. Return the chicken to the skillet and stir well. Taste for salt and pepper. Top off with the pecans before serving.

NOTE:

Toast the pecans in a medium skillet over low heat for 5 to 7 minutes, stirring frequently, until browned on all sides and fragrant.

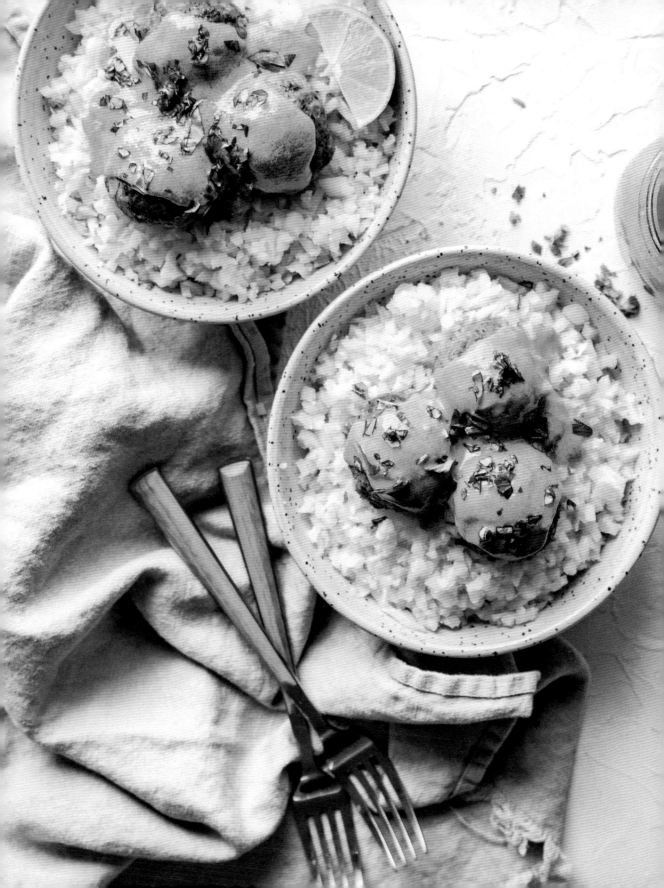

CHAPTER 6

main dishes

I AM BEYOND EXCITED FOR THIS MAIN DISH CHAPTER! You'll find so many fresh, exciting, and bold flavors here. My goal was to create recipes that you were going to want to come back to time and time again. Of course, I also wanted these dishes to be perfect for meal prep and something you could reheat and serve all week long if you wanted to. We are a family that loves leftovers, and I'm no stranger to reheating some salmon burgers and eating them alongside a big breakfast salad or with some breakfast potatoes.

In this chapter, you'll find those salmon burgers, along with Lamb & Beef Kofta, Crackling Pork Belly, and Flautas Casserole. Does all that sound absolutely fabulous? That's because it is! In this chapter, in particular, I've really drawn influences from myriad cultures around the world. Though we primarily cook Asian-style cuisine in our house, I found myself completely engulfed in so many other worlds when coming up with these main dishes. I hope you love them all!

◀ The Best Curry Meatballs, page 125

PREP TIME:
20 minutes
COOK TIME:
40 minutes
YIELD:
4 servings

DAIRY / GRAIN

Avocado oil or melted
   coconut oil
1½ pounds (680 g) boneless,
   skinless chicken thighs
1 cup (240 ml) filtered water
2 tablespoons (8 g) dried
   oregano
2 teaspoons (12 g) kosher
   salt, plus more to taste
1 teaspoon (2 g) black
   pepper, plus more to taste
¼ cup (40 g) thinly sliced
   scallions
3 tablespoons (45 g) cream
   cheese
3 tablespoons (45 ml) Clean
   Paleo Mayo (page 176)
2 tablespoons (30 ml) hot
   sauce
8 to 12 grain-free or corn
   tortillas
1½ cups (350 ml) 15-Minute
   Blender Salsa (page 179),
   plus more for serving
   (optional)
¾ cup (90 g) shredded white
   cheddar cheese
Chopped cilantro, for garnish

flautas casserole

I have a really good friend named Jeanette who is seriously one of the best cooks in the world. She has a way of making anything taste so comforting and beyond delicious. She once came to my house to make me flautas (which are tortillas that are filled, rolled, and fried), and I nearly lost my mind. I thought it would be a fabulous idea to pair flautas with salsa and cheese and turn the whole thing into a baked casserole. Even better, I cook the chicken thighs in the Instant Pot first so that they're super tender. This dish is so homey and inviting, and it tastes out of this world. I cannot wait for you to share it with your loved ones!

1 Preheat the oven to 375°F (190°C) and adjust the oven rack to the middle position. Lightly spray or brush an 8 x 8-inch (20.5 x 20.5 cm) or 9 x 7-inch (23 x 18 cm) baking dish with the oil.

2 Put the thighs into the Instant Pot. Add the water, oregano, salt, and pepper.

3 Set the Instant Pot to Sealing and pressure cook on Manual High pressure for 12 minutes. Let the pressure release naturally for 10 minutes, then carefully quick release the pressure.

4 Transfer the chicken from the liquid into a large bowl and shred with two forks. Add the scallions, cream cheese, mayo, and hot sauce. Mix everything together. Taste for additional salt and pepper.

5 Spray or brush oil onto the tortillas so they do not rip when being stuffed with the chicken mixture. Spread about ¼ cup (56 g) of the chicken mixture onto a tortilla. Carefully roll it into a log and place it into the casserole dish, seam-side down. Repeat until you've used all the filling. Cover the flautas with the salsa and cheese.

6 Bake until the cheese is glistening and the tortillas look cooked, 15 to 18 minutes. Sprinkle with cilantro. Serve with extra salsa, if you'd like, and enjoy hot.

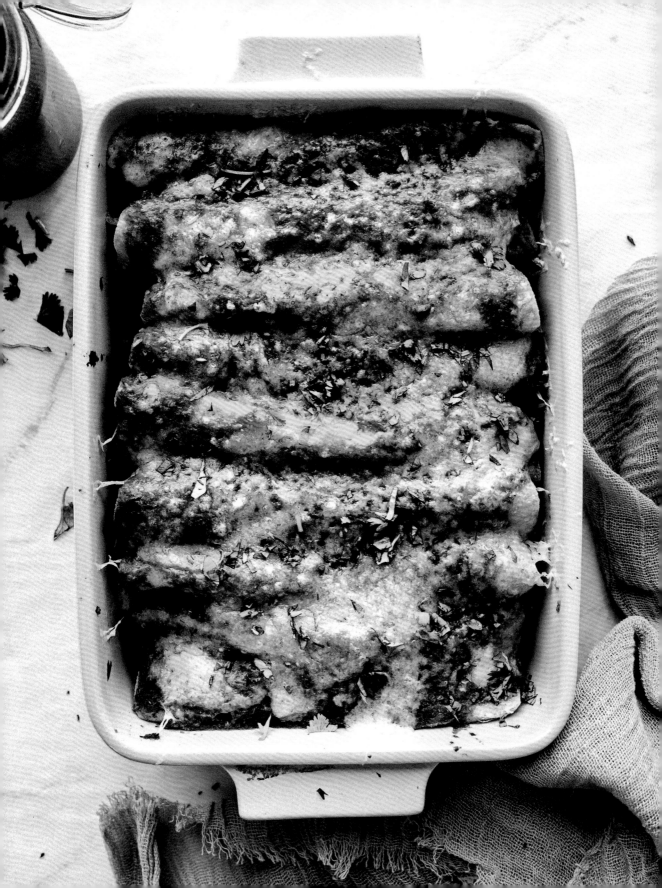

PREP TIME:
15 minutes

COOK TIME:
20 minutes

YIELD:
6 to 8 servings

lamb & beef kofta with tahini sauce

SAUCE
⅔ cup (160 g) tahini paste
   (see Notes)
½ cup (120 ml) filtered water
2½ tablespoons (37 ml)
   fresh lemon juice
2 cloves garlic, crushed
½ teaspoon lemon zest
¼ teaspoon kosher salt
Pinch of black pepper

KOFTA
1 pound (450 g) grass-fed
   85/15 ground beef
1 pound (450 g) ground lamb
2½ tablespoons (37 ml) harissa
2 teaspoons (4 g) lemon zest
2 cloves garlic, minced
1 teaspoon (2.3 g) ground
   cinnamon
1 teaspoon (1.8 g) ground
   ginger
1 teaspoon (2.5 g) ground cumin
1 teaspoon (6 g) kosher salt

8 metal skewers (see Notes)
Chopped fresh parsley,
   for garnish

This dish brings me back to my heritage in such a delightful fashion. I traveled to Israel in 2008, and to this day, it is definitely the most memorable trip of my life. A lot of that has to do with the experiences I had and the memories I created in relation to the food we ate. I am pretty sure I ate my body weight in kofta and tahini, so this recipe is an homage to that magical time.

1   Preheat the oven to 350°F (180°C). Line a rimmed baking sheet with parchment paper or aluminum foil.

2   To make the sauce, in a medium bowl, whisk together the tahini, water, lemon juice, garlic, lemon zest, salt, and pepper until well combined. You may need to add another tablespoon or two (15 to 30 ml) of water; the sauce should be thick, but pourable. Set aside.

3   To make the kofta, in a large bowl, combine the ground beef and lamb with the harissa, lemon zest, garlic, cinnamon, ginger, cumin, and salt. Using your hands, mix well to distribute the ingredients evenly.

4   Using about ¼ cup (32 g) of the mixture, carefully shape the meat into sausage link–size cylinders around each skewer. Set each skewer in a single layer on the prepared baking sheet.

5   Bake until the meat is cooked through but not overdone, 15 to 20 minutes. You can carefully cut through one of them and check to see if the meat is done in the center. A little bit of pink is fine.

6   Serve the kofta with the tahini sauce, garnished with the parsley.

NOTES:

Look for a tahini paste that is pourable and not too thick/chunky.

If you do not have skewers, you could make these into meatballs. Serve them (or the kofta) on a bed of your favorite rice.

PREP TIME:
5 minutes

COOK TIME:
2 hours 10 minutes

YIELD:
4 to 6 servings

SWEETENER

2 pounds (900 g) pork belly (see Notes)

1 tablespoon (18 g) kosher salt

1½ teaspoons (3 g) black pepper

2½ tablespoons (22.5 g) coconut sugar (see Notes)

2½ tablespoons (37 ml) fish sauce

NOTES:

You can purchase pork belly rolled into medallions or a thick slab. If it is rolled, be sure to unroll it and lay it on the wire rack with the thickest piece of fat facing up.

Run the coconut sugar through a food processor or spice/coffee grinder to turn it into more of a powder first. That will help it dissolve better in the fish sauce.

crackling pork belly

This crispy yet succulent pork belly is going to transport you to Asia, and you aren't going to want to come back, that's for sure. The top layer is crispy and chewy while the rest of the meat is soft and beyond juicy. There are only five ingredients, and it's mostly hands-off cooking. Your house is going to smell so good! It tastes best coming right out of the oven, but it's great as leftovers throughout the week—just be sure to reheat it in the pan to crisp it up again and so the fat can break down. Serve it with rice or use it to top off your favorite salad for extra protein.

1   Preheat the oven to its high broiling point and adjust the oven rack to the top third position. Place a wire rack inside a baking sheet, lined with aluminum foil if desired.

2   Lay the belly out onto a big cutting board, fat side up.

3   Using a paring knife, score the skin of the belly without cutting into the meat underneath.

4   Sprinkle generously with the salt and pepper. Make sure you get all the seasoning into the crevices of the fat. Really work it in there with your fingertips.

5   Place the belly on the wire rack and broil until the skin begins to crackle. Make sure you turn it every 5 minutes so it crackles/cooks evenly. This will take anywhere from 7 to 10 minutes total.

6   After the top is crispy, lower the oven heat to 275°F (140°C).

7   Bake for 1 hour and pull out the pork. Mix the coconut sugar and fish sauce together. Brush it on the belly, again making sure it gets into all the nooks and crannies. Stick the pork back into the oven, rotated 180 degrees, and bake for 1 hour more.

8   Slice and serve with your favorite type of rice, inside of a taco, or on top of a salad.

PREP TIME:
10 minutes +
marinating time

COOK TIME:
20 minutes

YIELD:
6 to 8 servings

clean paleo steak fajitas

These steak fajitas are quick to make and full of so much flavor. In fact, you'll only need one pan to make this healthy and filling meal. If you can get your hands on a cast-iron pan, do; then you'll get the full experience of this fabulous dish. Either way, this recipe is great for meal prep all week long, and I've been known to grab a few slices of the cold flank steak to throw on salads, too. Absolutely delicious!

MARINADE

⅓ cup (80 ml) coconut aminos

¼ cup (60 ml) avocado oil

2 limes, 1 zested, 2 juiced

1½ teaspoons (3.8 g) ground cumin

1½ teaspoons (9 g) kosher salt, plus more to season

1 teaspoon (1.2 g) crushed red pepper flakes

¾ teaspoon garlic powder

¾ teaspoon onion powder

Black pepper, plus more to season

1½ to 2 pounds (680 to 900 g) flank steak

VEGGIES

¼ cup (60 ml) chicken bone broth or low-sodium chicken broth

4 medium zucchini, sliced

4 bell peppers (any color), thinly sliced

1 yellow onion, sliced

1   To make the marinade, in a small bowl, whisk together the coconut aminos, oil, lime zest and juice, cumin, salt, red pepper flakes, garlic powder, onion powder, and a large pinch of black pepper. Transfer the marinade to a gallon-size (4 L) resealable plastic bag and add the flank steak.

2   Press out any excess air and close the bag. Massage the meat thoroughly with your fingers so the marinade is evenly incorporated. Let it marinate in the refrigerator for at least 1 hour, but take it out again 30 minutes before you want to cook it.

3   Heat a large cast-iron pan over medium-high heat. Remove the flank steak from the bag and place on a cutting board. Reserve the marinade. Generously sprinkle the steak with salt and black pepper.

4   Gently place the steak into the pan and cook until a brown crust has formed, 4½ to 5 minutes. Flip over and cook for another 4½ to 5 minutes (see Notes). Remove the steak from the pan and let rest for 10 minutes with foil tented over it.

5   While the steak is resting, cook the vegetables (see Notes). Add the bone broth to the skillet and scrape up the brown bits left over in the pan. Add the zucchini, bell peppers, and onion and cook until softened, 8 to 10 minutes. Add the reserved marinade about halfway through. Bring to a boil, then lower the heat and let the marinade reduce.

6   Divide the vegetables among plates. Slice the steak against the grain and layer on top.

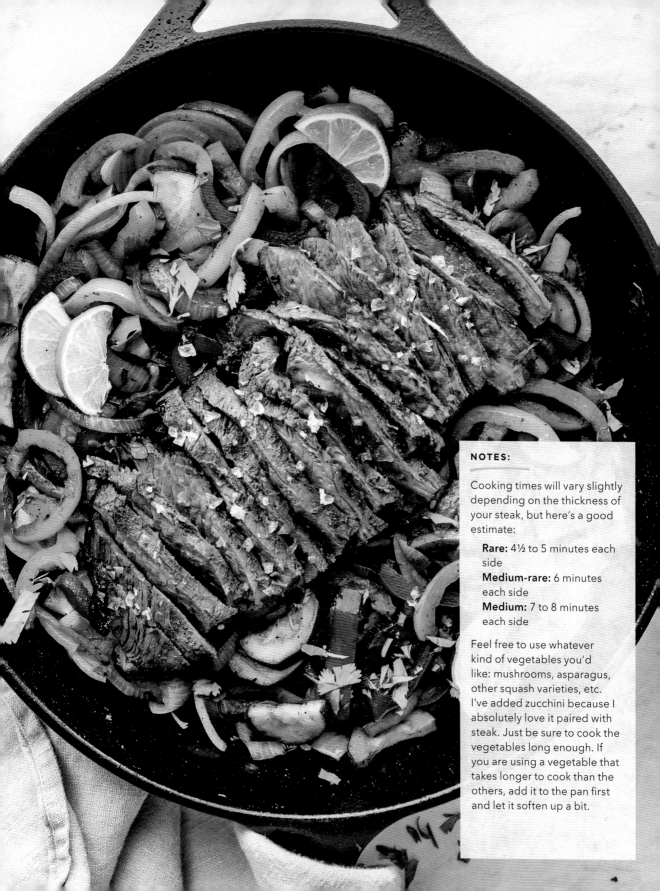

NOTES:

Cooking times will vary slightly depending on the thickness of your steak, but here's a good estimate:

Rare: 4½ to 5 minutes each side

Medium-rare: 6 minutes each side

Medium: 7 to 8 minutes each side

Feel free to use whatever kind of vegetables you'd like: mushrooms, asparagus, other squash varieties, etc. I've added zucchini because I absolutely love it paired with steak. Just be sure to cook the vegetables long enough. If you are using a vegetable that takes longer to cook than the others, add it to the pan first and let it soften up a bit.

PREP TIME:
15 minutes

COOK TIME:
90 minutes

YIELD:
6 servings

GRAIN / DAIRY

pork ragú with polenta

RAGÚ

2½ pounds (1.13 kg) pork shoulder/Boston butt (see Note, page 110)

Kosher salt, to taste

Black pepper, to taste

1½ tablespoons (22 ml) avocado oil

1 small yellow onion, diced

6 cloves garlic, minced

1 cup (240 ml) low-sodium chicken or bone broth

2 tablespoons (32 g) tomato paste

6 sprigs thyme

2 sprigs rosemary

2 bay leaves

1 can (14 ounces [396 g]) whole peeled tomatoes (San Marzanos are great!)

POLENTA

8 cups (1.9 L) filtered water

2 teaspoons (12 g) kosher salt

Scant 2 cups (320 g) polenta corn grits

6 tablespoons (85 g) grass-fed butter or ghee

1 cup (90 g) finely grated Parmesan cheese, plus more for garnish

Chopped fresh parsley, for garnish

This dish gives me serious authentic Italian vibes—but without too much time in the kitchen. Prepare the polenta while the pork shoulder is in the pressure cooker, and everything will be done at about the same time. If you want to impress with a bomb dinner party, this is the dish you should make. It's luscious, hearty, and absolutely phenomenal!

1 To make the ragú, cut the pork shoulder into 3 chunks. Pat very dry with a paper towel and sprinkle liberally with salt and pepper.

2 Turn the Instant Pot to Sauté and heat for 1 minute. Add the oil and heat for another minute. Brown all the pieces of pork on each side, about 10 minutes total. Transfer to a plate. Discard any burnt pieces in the pot.

3 Add the onion and a pinch of salt. Sauté, stirring frequently, until soft and caramelization begins, about 5 minutes. Add the garlic and cook for another minute, stirring frequently.

4 Deglaze the pot with the broth, scraping off the browned bits from the bottom. Add the tomato paste, thyme, rosemary, and bay leaves. Cook for a few minutes, stirring often, until the liquid reduces by about half.

5 Add the pork back to the pot, along with its juices, and the tomatoes (with their juice), squishing the tomatoes as you add them. Cover and set the valve to Sealing. Cook for 35 minutes on Manual High pressure.

6 When finished, let the pressure release naturally for about 15 minutes, then cover the valve with a kitchen towel and switch it to Venting. While the pressure is releasing, start the polenta.

(continued)

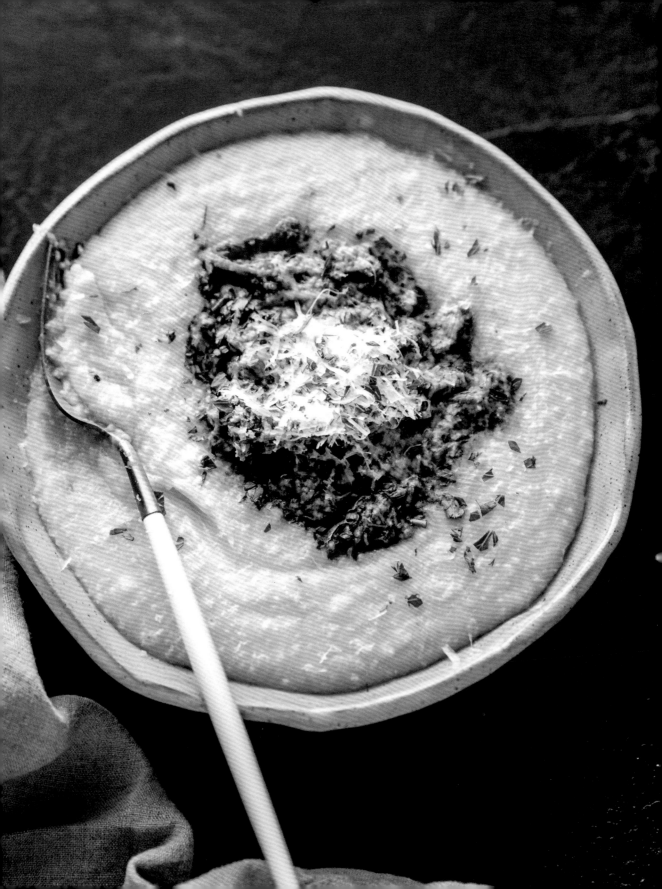

7 To make the polenta, add the water and salt to a large saucepan. Bring to a low boil. Slowly pour in the polenta, whisking constantly. Once there are no lumps, reduce the heat to low.

8 Whisking frequently, cook until it begins to slightly thicken, 2 to 3 minutes. Cover and cook for 25 minutes, whisking every 5 minutes. When it becomes too thick to whisk, use a wooden spoon instead.

9 In between stirs of the polenta, finish the pork. Open the pot, and if there is a top layer of fat in there, feel free to remove it with a spoon. Transfer the pork pieces to a cutting board and shred with two forks. Remove the herbs and bay leaves from the pot. Add the shredded pork back in and stir well.

10 Once the polenta looks very creamy and the individual grains are tender, it is done. Turn off the heat and gently stir in the butter. Add the Parmesan and stir until melted. Cover and let stand for a few minutes to thicken. Stir again and taste for seasoning. It needs to be served immediately before it begins to "set."

11 Serve the pork over the polenta and garnish with more Parmesan and chopped parsley.

12 Polenta can be stored as leftovers in an airtight container in the refrigerator. To reheat and rehydrate, add to a small pot with a few tablespoons of water and some butter. Cook over low heat for a few minutes, stirring frequently.

PREP TIME:
5 minutes +
marinating time
COOK TIME:
10 minutes
YIELD:
6 servings

vietnamese lemongrass chicken

¼ cup (60 ml) fresh
   lime juice
3 tablespoons (45 ml)
   fish sauce
3 tablespoons (14.4 g)
   chopped fresh lemongrass
   (see Note)
4 tablespoons (60 ml)
   avocado oil, divided
6 cloves garlic
1 shallot, halved
1 tablespoon (15 ml)
   coconut aminos
1 teaspoon (6 g) kosher salt
2 pounds (900 g) boneless,
   skinless chicken thighs

Are you ready for some seriously flavorful and authentic-tasting lemongrass chicken? My husband is Vietnamese, and he's really particular about how Vietnamese dishes should taste (especially when I try my hand at them!). This lemongrass chicken absolutely gets his stamp of approval. The succulent, umami-packed chicken thighs are going to make your taste buds go nuts, I promise you that. They are so easy to make and taste wonderful with rice or cauliflower rice, and your favorite vegetables. I love making a big batch to have on hand throughout the week to pair with different sides I whip up.

1 In a blender, combine the lime juice, fish sauce, lemongrass, 2 table-spoons (30 ml) of the oil, garlic, shallot, coconut aminos, and salt. Blend on high speed until creamy throughout.

2 Place the chicken thighs in a gallon-size (4 L) resealable plastic bag with the marinade. Make sure it can lie flat in the refrigerator so the marinade is evenly dispersed.

3 After at least 1 hour (but up to overnight), remove the chicken from the refrigerator. Heat a large nonstick skillet over medium-high heat. Add the remaining 2 tablespoons (30 ml) oil and remove the chicken from the marinade (discard the marinade). You may need to work in two batches, depending on the size of your skillet.

4 Cook the chicken until brown on each side and cooked through to 165°F (74°C), 4 to 5 minutes per side. Serve hot.

NOTE:

If you cannot find fresh lemongrass, buy a lemongrass paste, usually found near the herbs in the produce section, and use the same amount.

PREP TIME:
10 minutes +
chill time

COOK TIME:
10 minutes

YIELD:
6 burgers

crispy salmon patty burgers

1½ pounds (680 g) skinless, center-cut salmon fillet, finely chopped

½ cup (120 ml) Paleo Mayo (page 176)

½ cup (25 g) fresh cilantro, chopped

½ cup (25 g) fresh mint, chopped

2 tablespoons (30 ml) fish sauce

2 tablespoons (30 ml) hot sauce

1 medium shallot, minced

3 cloves garlic, minced

1 tablespoon (6 g) minced fresh ginger

½ teaspoon finely grated lemon zest

1 teaspoon (6 g) kosher salt

½ teaspoon black pepper

1½ cups (180 g) almond flour

2 tablespoons (30 ml) avocado oil or ghee, divided

12 leaves butter lettuce

6 slices tomato

1 batch Lemon Aioli (page 68)

These salmon patty burgers are beyond delicious, as they are full of fresh ingredients and paired with the best creamy, lemony spread ever. Get ready for a flavor explosion in your mouth. Oh, and they taste good all week long, so they are a perfect addition to your meal prep.

1 In the bowl of a food processor, pulse the salmon a few seconds at a time until it is minced. Be careful not to turn it into a total puree. Set aside.

2 In a large bowl, mix together the mayo, cilantro, mint, fish sauce, hot sauce, shallot, garlic, ginger, and lemon zest. Mix until well combined. Add the salt and pepper

3 Transfer the minced salmon to the bowl. Give everything a nice stir. Add the almond flour, ½ cup (60 g) at a time, and combine thoroughly.

4 Line a small baking sheet with parchment paper. With lightly oiled hands, form the salmon mixture into 6 even patties, by rolling each into a ball first and then flattening with your hands. Add the patties to the baking sheet and cover with plastic wrap. Refrigerate for 2 to 6 hours.

5 Heat 1 tablespoon (15 ml) of the oil in a large nonstick skillet for 1 minute. Cook 3 salmon patties at a time until golden brown, 3 to 4 minutes. Flip and cook for another 3 minutes. They should be golden on the outside and barely cooked in the center. Remove to a plate and repeat with the remaining oil and salmon patties.

6 Build the burgers by layering a salmon patty on two butter lettuce leaves. Top off with a fresh tomato slice and some lemon aioli. Serve right away.

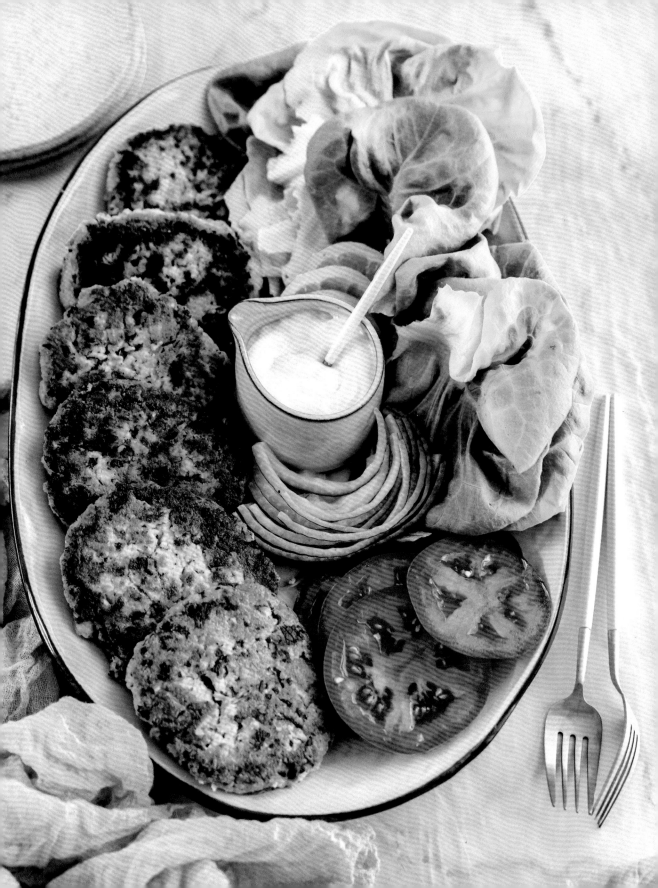

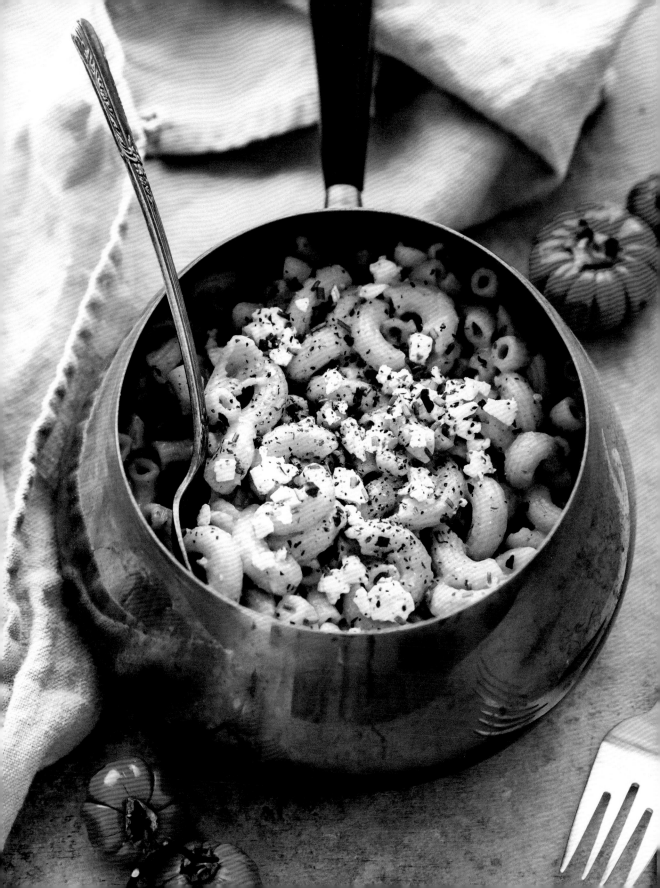

PREP TIME:
5 minutes

COOK TIME:
20 minutes

YIELD:
4 servings

GRAIN / DAIRY

rice pasta with pumpkin alfredo

1 teaspoon (6 g) kosher salt, plus more to taste

8 ounces (140 g) rice pasta (see Note)

1 batch Pumpkin Alfredo Sauce (page 180)

Black pepper, to taste

¼ cup (60 g) sheep's milk feta cheese, crumbled (optional)

¼ cup (40 g) finely chopped fresh chives

Crushed red pepper flakes, to taste

It's no secret I'm a carnivore through and through. However, once in a blue moon, I come up with a really delicious vegetarian main dish that is something to get really excited about. This rice pasta with pumpkin alfredo is one of those recipes. You may be thinking: "Pumpkin alfredo? What? Why?" Once you try it, though, there will be no more questions. It's going to taste warm, comforting, and reminiscent of all the coziest and best feelings. Thank me after!

1 In a large pot, bring 4 quarts (4 L) of water to a boil over high heat. Add 1 teaspoon (6 g) salt.

2 Add the pasta and stir gently for 3 to 5 seconds.

3 Maintain a rolling boil, stirring occasionally, and cook until your desired tenderness, 10 to 12 minutes, depending on the shape and size of the pasta you bought. (Follow the cooking instructions on the box.)

4 Meanwhile, warm the alfredo sauce in a medium saucepan over medium heat.

5 Drain the pasta and rinse well with cold water.

6 Transfer the pasta to a large bowl. Add the sauce and toss to coat well. (You might need less than the whole batch.) Taste for additional salt and add pepper, if desired.

7 Top with the feta (if using), chives, and red pepper flakes before serving.

NOTE:

I recommend 8 ounces (226 g) of pasta because depending on how saucy you like your pasta, a 12-ounce (340 g) box might be too much.

PREP TIME:
20 minutes
COOK TIME:
15 minutes
YIELD:
6 servings

kung pao chicken

CHICKEN
1 large egg
¼ cup (60 ml) coconut
  aminos
1 teaspoon (3 g) arrowroot
  flour
½ teaspoon garlic powder
¼ teaspoon onion powder
¼ teaspoon kosher salt
1½ pounds (680 g) boneless,
  skinless chicken thighs,
  cut into bite-size chunks
3 tablespoons (45 ml)
  avocado oil, divided

STIR-FRY SAUCE
¼ cup (60 ml) coconut
  aminos
1½ teaspoons (7.5 ml)
  rice vinegar
1 heaping teaspoon (16 g)
  tomato paste
1 teaspoon (5 ml) toasted
  sesame oil
½ teaspoon arrowroot flour

AROMATICS
6 cloves garlic, thinly sliced
1½ tablespoons (9 g) finely
  chopped fresh ginger
3 scallion bulbs, chopped
  (reserve greens for garnish)
6 dried red chile peppers
  (see Note)
1 fresh Thai chile, finely
  chopped
1 tablespoon (5 g) Sichuan
  peppercorns
Kosher salt, to taste

Here's a healthy, quick, and easy version of one of the most popular Chinese stir-fries. It's packed with all the flavor while remaining nutrient dense and Clean Paleo compliant—and you won't feel bloated or uneasy after having a bowl, even if you pair it with lots of cauliflower rice. The aromatics are an absolute must to infuse such powerful flavor in such a short amount of time. The key to making this fast is to get the chicken into the marinade, then get all the other ingredients ready to go before you even turn on the stove. So the next time somebody mentions take-out, you'll likely chime in, "No, I got this. We're making kung pao chicken here tonight!"

1 To make the chicken, in a small bowl, whisk together the egg, coconut aminos, arrowroot flour, garlic powder, onion powder, and salt.

2 Place the chicken thighs in a shallow but long glass dish. Pour the marinade over the top. Make sure the chicken pieces are fully submerged in the marinade. Refrigerate for 15 to 20 minutes while you prepare the other ingredients.

3 Meanwhile, make the stir-fry sauce by whisking together the coconut aminos, vinegar, tomato paste, oil, and arrowroot flour in a small bowl. Set aside.

4 Preheat a large stainless-steel skillet over medium-high heat. After about 1 minute, add 1½ tablespoons (22 ml) of the avocado oil. Add the chicken and panfry the pieces in a single even layer until they begin to crisp up and turn golden brown, 5 to 6 minutes. Flip them over and cook for another minute. Remove from the pan and set aside.

5 With the skillet still over medium-high heat, add the remaining 1½ tablespoons (23 ml) avocado oil. Add the aromatics and sprinkle with a bit of salt. Sauté just until fragrant, 10 to 15 seconds.

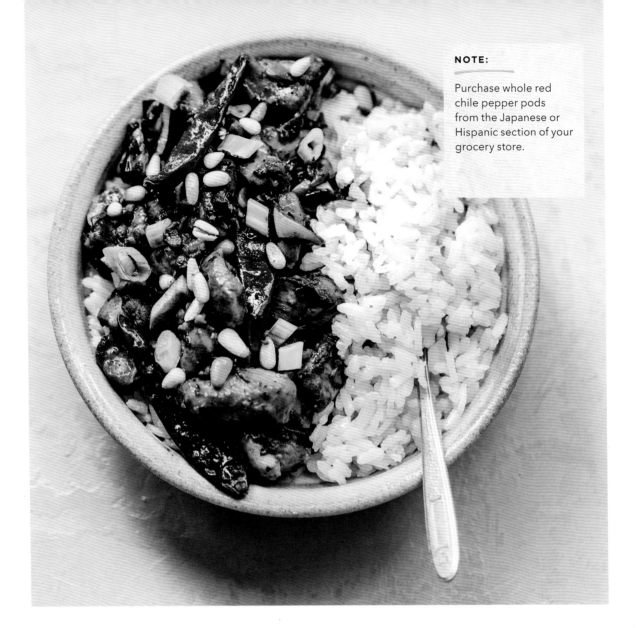

NOTE:

Purchase whole red chile pepper pods from the Japanese or Hispanic section of your grocery store.

GARNISH
Sliced scallion greens
Toasted pine nuts
Toasted sesame oil
Coconut aminos

Immediately add the stir-fry sauce. Quickly mix everything together to completely coat the aromatics with the sauce. Add the chicken back to the skillet. Stir well to fully combine the chicken, aromatics, and sauce. Once the chicken is cooked through, 3 to 5 more minutes, remove from the heat.

6 Serve immediately with chopped scallion greens and toasted pine nuts. Season with extra sesame oil and coconut aminos according to your taste preference!

PREP TIME:
5 minutes

COOK TIME:
6 minutes +
rest time

YIELD:
2 servings

best cast-iron ribeye

1 ribeye steak (approximately
1 pound [453 g])
Avocado oil
2 teaspoons (5 g) Best Steak
Rub (page 185)
2 tablespoons (30 ml)
grass-fed butter or ghee

I've got a recipe for a steak that will turn out perfectly every time. With a really incredible dry rub, the right pan, and the right fat, you are going to be making the best steaks of your life. Get ready, though, because your friends and family will be wanting you to make your fabulous steaks every time you all get together. It's not much of a burden to take on if they agree to call you "Steak Master"!

1 Pull the steak from the refrigerator about 30 minutes before you plan to start cooking and place it on a cutting board. Pat both sides dry with a paper towel.

2 Lightly brush or spray both sides of the steak with avocado oil.

3 Sprinkle 1 teaspoon (2.5 g) of the seasoning on each side of the steak.

4 Add the butter or ghee to a cast-iron pan and heat for 2 minutes over high heat. Add the steak to the pan and set a timer for 3 minutes (see Notes).

5 Flip the steak over and turn the heat to medium-high. Cook for another 3 minutes.

6 Transfer the steak to a cutting board or plate and tent aluminum foil over the top. After 10 minutes, slice and serve.

NOTES:

Cooking times will vary slightly depending on the thickness of your steak, but here's a good estimate:

Rare: 3 minutes per side
Medium-rare: 3 to 4 minutes per side
Medium: 5 to 7 minutes per side
Medium-well: 8 to 10 minutes per side

You can also use this recipe with different steak cuts. Simply adjust the cooking times depending on the thickness of the meat.

PREP TIME:
20 minutes

COOK TIME:
10 minutes

YIELD:
6 servings

SWEETENER

2 tablespoons (30 ml) ghee or avocado oil

2 pounds (900 g) grass-fed 85/15 or 90/10 ground beef

¼ cup (12.5 g) fresh cilantro, coarsely chopped

¼ cup (60 ml) coconut aminos

3 tablespoons (45 ml) honey

2 tablespoons (30 ml) toasted sesame oil

8 cloves garlic, minced

2 tablespoons (30 ml) fish sauce

1 tablespoon (15 ml) rice vinegar

1 teaspoon (1.2 g) crushed red pepper flakes

Romaine hearts or butter lettuce, for wrapping

1 batch Triple-C Sauce (page 182)

easy beef lettuce wraps

This low-carb dish is going to leave you feeling all kinds of fine, and you may break out in song and dance, too. The Triple-C Sauce that is drizzled on top really highlights and heightens the Asian-inspired flavors of the ground beef. Grab these for a quick and easy to-go lunch!

1 In a large skillet over medium-high heat, melt the ghee. Once the pan is hot, add the ground beef.

2 Cook the meat, continuously stirring to break it up, until it is brown throughout, 5 to 6 minutes. Remove from the heat, strain the fat, and transfer the meat to a large bowl.

3 Stir in the cilantro, coconut aminos, honey, sesame oil, garlic, fish sauce, vinegar, and red pepper flakes.

4 Assemble the wraps. In a lettuce leaf, spoon out a few tablespoons of ground beef and top off with a few drizzles of the sauce. Serve warm (but they're also great cold!).

PREP TIME:
10 minutes

COOK TIME:
10 minutes

YIELD:
4 bowls

fish taco bowls

FISH

1½ pounds (680 g) cod, cut into 2 fillets

1 tablespoon (15 ml) fresh lime juice

2 teaspoons (5.2 g) chili powder

½ teaspoon ground cumin

½ teaspoon onion powder

½ teaspoon garlic powder

½ teaspoon kosher salt

Black pepper, to taste

1 tablespoon (15 ml) avocado oil

BOWLS

4 large handfuls mixed greens or lettuce

3 bags (12 ounces [340 g]) cauliflower rice, cooked according to package directions

1 batch Creamy Cashew Ranch Dip (page XX), made chipotle according to Notes

2 avocados, sliced, for topping

1 cup (150 g) cherry tomatoes, halved, for topping

Lime wedges, for topping

¼ cup (40 g) sliced scallions, for topping

1 jalapeño, sliced, for topping

These paleo fish taco bowls are such a well-balanced meal, they will fill you right up. They're made with delicious panfried white fish, lots of veggies, and cauliflower rice, topped off with a creamy cashew chipotle sauce—make this first, even the day before, since the cashews need time to soak. Sign me up for this easy, nutritious, and delicious meal, please! Be prepared, though, because you are going to go back for seconds.

1 To make the fish, rinse the fish fillets with cold water and pat dry very well. Set on a cutting board.

2 In a small bowl, whisk together the lime juice, chili powder, cumin, onion powder, garlic powder, salt, and a few grinds of black pepper. Using a brush or your hands, cover the fillets evenly with the marinade.

3 Heat a large skillet over medium heat for 1 minute. Add the oil and cook both fillets until they are flaky when touched with a fork, about 3 minutes on the first side and 2 minutes on the other. Remove the skillet from the heat.

4 To make the bowls, layer some leafy greens or lettuce leaves in a bowl with the cooked cauliflower rice. Top off with the flaked fish, the cashew ranch, and your desired toppings. Serve right away.

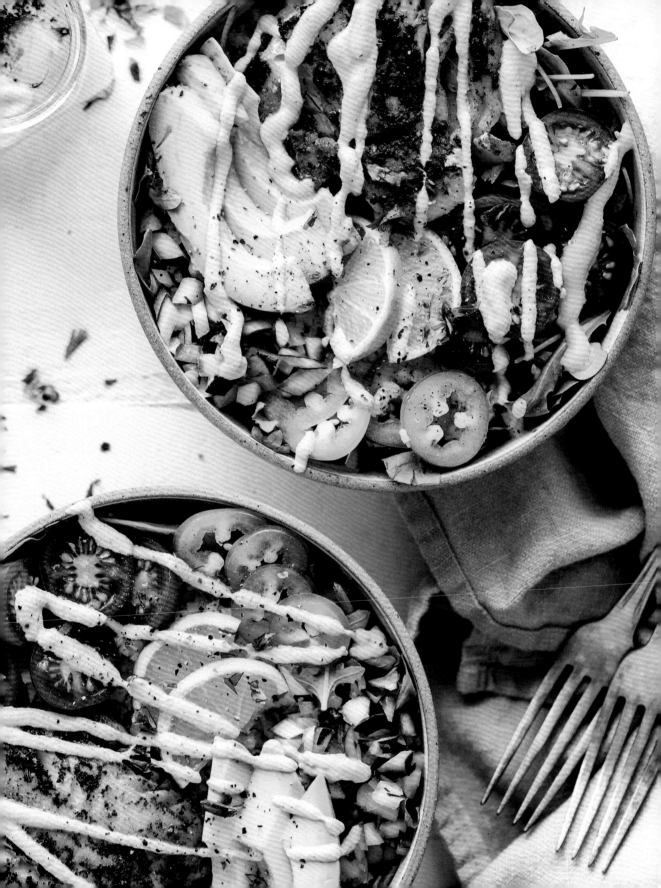

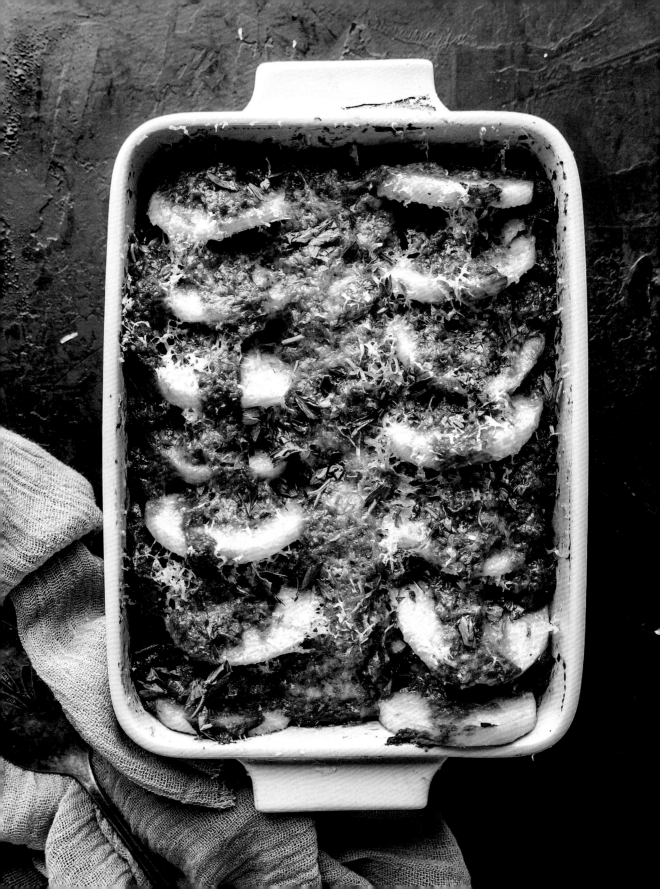

PREP TIME:
10 minutes

COOK TIME:
25 minutes

YIELD:
4 to 6 servings

GRAIN / DAIRY

baked polenta with sausage & artichoke hearts

2 tablespoons (30 ml) avocado oil

½ white onion, diced large

1 pound (450 g) Italian sausage, casings removed

4 cloves garlic, minced

1 cup (150 g) artichoke hearts in water, drained and coarsely chopped

Kosher salt, to taste

Black pepper, to taste

1½ pounds (680 g) polenta, prepared in a tube, sliced into ½-inch (1.3 cm) rounds

⅓ cup (80 ml) chicken broth

1½ cups (350 ml) red sauce (marinara sauce)

¼ cup (22 g) grated Parmesan cheese (optional)

¼ cup (12.5 g) fresh parsley, chopped

Are you ready for something that tastes like it came straight out of an authentic Italian restaurant? Well, here it is. This baked polenta dish pretty much gives me lasagna vibes, but it's actually super light. It's the perfect weeknight meal and tastes delicious when reheated as leftovers.

1 Preheat the oven to 400°F (200°C) and adjust the oven rack to the middle position.

2 In a large skillet over medium heat, add the oil. After 1 minute, add the onion. Cook until soft, stirring frequently, about 5 minutes.

3 Add the sausage and cook, while breaking up the meat with a wooden spoon, until browned, 7 to 8 minutes. Add the garlic and cook for about 1 minute, stirring frequently, until fragrant.

4 Remove the skillet from the heat and stir in the artichoke hearts and a big pinch of salt and pepper.

5 Transfer the mixture to a 2-quart (2 L) baking dish and nestle the polenta rounds in it. Pour the broth evenly on top of the dish. Cover with the red sauce and cheese, if using.

6 Bake until the polenta is glistening and the cheese has melted, 20 to 25 minutes. Sprinkle with the parsley and serve warm.

PREP TIME:
10 minutes

COOK TIME:
40 minutes

YIELD:
20 meatballs

cauliflower rice meatballs

MEATBALLS
4 strips bacon, diced
1½ pounds (680 g) grass-fed lean ground beef
1 cup (150 g) cauliflower rice
⅓ cup (50 g) finely diced yellow onion
¼ cup (60 ml) coconut cream (see Note)
1½ teaspoons (9 g) kosher salt
¼ teaspoon ground ginger
1 large egg, whisked

SAUCE
½ cup (120 ml) plus 2 tablespoons (30 ml) coconut aminos
¼ cup (60 ml) plus 1½ tablespoons (22 ml) filtered water, divided
1 tablespoon (15 ml) apple cider vinegar
1½ teaspoons (7.5 ml) extra virgin olive oil
1 teaspoon (2 g) minced fresh ginger
½ teaspoon garlic powder
1 tablespoon (8 g) arrowroot flour

NOTE:

To make coconut cream, refrigerate a can of full-fat coconut milk overnight and scoop off the top layer that separates. If you can purchase coconut cream, make sure it has 10 to 12 grams of fat.

Is there anything better than adding a nutrient-dense veggie to a meat-centric dish and fooling the crowd? Nope. This is especially true when it comes to getting nutrients in for your kids. These cauliflower rice meatballs, rich with crispy bacon and coconut cream, are paired with a wonderfully zesty sauce. They are absolutely perfect for meal prep and taste delicious when reheated. Serve them over veggie noodles to round out the meal.

1 Preheat the oven to 350°F (180°C) and adjust the oven rack to the middle position. Line a baking sheet with parchment paper.

2 To make the meatballs, in a skillet over medium to medium-high heat, cook the bacon until crispy, about 5 minutes. Transfer to a paper towel–lined plate and let cool.

3 In a large mixing bowl, combine the ground beef, cauliflower, onion, coconut cream, salt, and ginger. Mix well with your hands, making sure everything is evenly dispersed. Add the egg and mix well again. Finally, add the bacon bits. Mix one last time.

4 Using a 2-tablespoon (30 ml) cookie scoop, scoop the meatballs and roll them between your palms to create a well-rounded ball. Transfer the meatballs to the prepared baking sheet.

5 Bake until the middles are just cooked through, 22 to 26 minutes.

6 Meanwhile, prepare the sauce. In a small saucepan, combine the coconut aminos, ¼ cup (60 ml) of the water, vinegar, oil, ginger, and garlic powder. Set over medium-low heat, stirring constantly, for 10 minutes.

7 In a small bowl, whisk together the remaining 1½ tablespoons (22 ml) water and arrowroot flour until smooth. Slowly whisk the arrowroot slurry into the sauce, cook for about 1 minute, then remove from the heat.

8 To serve, toss the meatballs with the sauce or serve them with the sauce on the side.

PREP TIME:
10 minutes

COOK TIME:
35 minutes

YIELD:
24 meatballs

the best curry meatballs

These meatballs are the perfect addition to your Clean Paleo weekly meal plan. Bring them with you to lunch atop a big and hearty salad, or enjoy them with a large bowl of cauliflower rice for dinner. Be sure to double up on the delicious, creamy sauce, too—you are going to wish you had extra to slather over all kinds of dinners throughout the week.

MEATBALLS

1 cup (150 g) coarsely chopped carrots

½ cup (75 g) cooked cauliflower rice

½ red onion, coarsely chopped

3 tablespoons (7.5 g) chopped fresh basil, plus more for garnish

6 cloves garlic

1½ limes, juiced

2 tablespoons (30 ml) coconut aminos

1 tablespoon (7 g) flaxseed meal

1½ teaspoons (1.8 g) ground ginger

1 teaspoon (2.5 g) ground cumin

½ teaspoon crushed red pepper flakes, plus more for garnish

½ teaspoon kosher salt

½ teaspoon black pepper

Splash of fish sauce

2 pounds (900 g) grass-fed 90/10 ground beef

CURRY SAUCE

1 can (13.5 ounces [380 ml]) full-fat coconut milk

3 tablespoons (45 g) cashew butter or almond butter

2 heaping tablespoons (30 g) red curry paste

2 limes, juiced

2 teaspoons (6 g) minced garlic

½ teaspoon ground ginger

2 tablespoons (16 g) arrowroot flour, whisked with 2 tablespoons (30 ml) filtered water (optional)

1 Preheat the oven to 375°F (190°C) and adjust the oven rack to the middle position. Line a baking sheet with parchment paper.

2 To make the meatballs, place the carrots, cauliflower rice, onion, basil, garlic, lime juice, coconut aminos, flax, ginger, cumin, red pepper flakes, salt, black pepper, and fish sauce in the bowl of a food processor. Pulse for 30 seconds or so until mixed well. Do not overprocess, or the mixture will become mushy! Add the beef and process a few more times.

3 Roll the mixture into 1½ to 2-inch (4 to 5 cm) balls and place them on the prepared baking sheet.

4 Bake for 20 minutes and rotate the sheet 180 degrees. Bake for another 10 to 15 minutes, until the meatballs have reached your desired doneness. I like mine cooked to a medium doneness, so I pull them out after 30 minutes total.

5 While the meatballs finish baking, prepare the sauce. In a medium saucepan, heat the coconut milk until it begins to simmer. Add the nut butter, curry paste, lime juice, garlic, and ginger and whisk well. Bring to a low boil, then turn the heat down to low. Let simmer and thicken for 10 to 15 minutes. If you like your sauce a bit thicker, you can add the optional arrowroot mixture.

6 Serve the meatballs covered with the curry sauce and garnished with fresh basil and red pepper flakes, if desired.

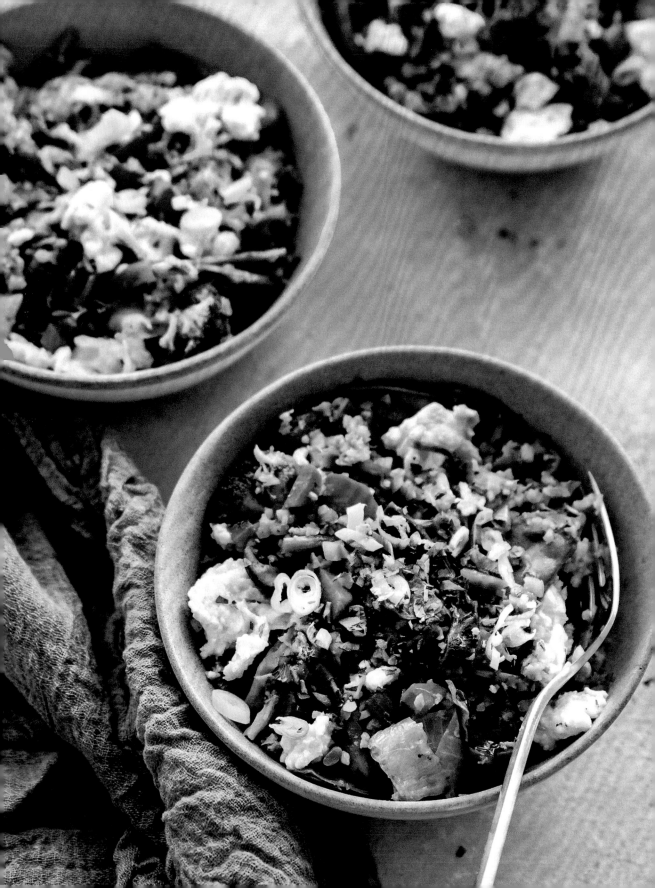

CHAPTER 7

side dishes

IS THERE ANYTHING WORSE than feeling completely unsatiated after finishing a meal? I think not. There have been numerous occasions where I had one of the best steaks ever, yet I was totally unimpressed with the accompaniments. Either the side dish wasn't substantial enough to hold up next to the meat or it just wasn't enough of a star in its own right. So in this chapter, I wanted to come up with a variety of side dishes that were going to leave you feeling really good about pairing them with *whatever* it is you're eating. These recipes are not an afterthought, as you will soon realize.

I've included a few of my favorites, like a spicy Buffalo Potato Salad, a bright Brussels Sprouts Slaw, and some Truffled Polenta Rounds that are beyond drool worthy. These side dishes easily hold their own and are not upstaged by any main course. Consider keeping a variety of these dishes ready-made in your refrigerator to pair with main dishes all week long. Your mouth (and stomach) will thank you.

◀ Umami-Filled Cauliflower Rice, page 136

PREP TIME:
20 minutes

COOK TIME:
10 minutes

YIELD:
6 to 8 servings

mediterranean cauliflower salad

DRESSING

⅓ cup (80 ml) red wine vinegar

⅓ cup (80 ml) extra virgin olive oil

2 tablespoons (30 ml) Lemon Aioli (page 68)

2 tablespoons (22 g) whole-grain mustard

1 teaspoon (1.4 g) dried thyme

½ teaspoon salt

SALAD

1 head cauliflower, cut into florets

12 ounces (340 g) haricots verts

1 cup (150 g) green olives, minced

1 cup (150 g) roasted red peppers, minced

½ red onion, finely diced

Handful fresh parsley, chopped

Handful fresh arugula

½ teaspoon black pepper

Salt, to taste

This Mediterranean cauliflower salad was inspired by a dish my grandma has always made for every single family gathering. She basically marinates a ton of my favorite vegetables in oil and vinegar and tops them off with fresh herbs and spices. Her rendition is very Italian, while mine rains down Mediterranean vibes. This would be great at a dinner party or simply alongside your breakfast, lunch, or dinner!

1　To make the dressing, in a small bowl, whisk together the vinegar, oil, aioli, mustard, thyme, and salt until thoroughly combined and no clumps of aioli remain. Set aside.

2　To make the salad, in a large frying pan, bring ¼ inch (6 mm) of water to a boil. Add the cauliflower and cover the pan. Steam until fork tender but not falling apart, about 6 minutes. Drain and set aside.

3　Meanwhile, bring 6 cups (1.4 L) of water to a boil in a deep pot and add the haricots verts. Boil for 6 minutes and drain. Cut into 1-inch (2.5 cm) segments and add to a large bowl, along with the cauliflower florets.

4　Add the olives, red peppers, onion, parsley, arugula, and black pepper and toss everything well.

5　Slowly pour in the dressing while mixing the salad. Taste for additional black pepper, adding salt if necessary.

PREP TIME:
15 minutes

COOK TIME:
60 minutes

YIELD:
8 servings

smashed potatoes with avocado aioli

- 2 pounds (900 g) Yukon gold or red potatoes
- 3 tablespoons (45 ml) avocado oil or extra virgin olive oil
- 1 teaspoon (3 g) garlic powder
- Kosher salt, to taste
- Black pepper, to taste
- ⅓ cup (5 g) fresh dill, minced
- 1 batch Avocado Aioli (page 179)

If you want to really please some folks, I highly encourage you to try out these smashed potatoes. They truly are potatoes that you get to smash before they go into the oven! The result is something truly magical: golden, crispy, but tender. And they're not just for dinner—eat them alongside breakfast or grab one for a snack. They're out of this world when paired with the creamy avocado aioli. (Prepare the aioli while the potatoes are roasting so it's at its greenest and freshest.)

1 Place the potatoes in a large pot and cover with cold water. Set on the stove over high heat. When the water begins to boil, reduce the heat to medium and boil until the potatoes are fork tender, 20 to 25 minutes.

2 While the potatoes boil, preheat the oven to 450°F (230°C) and lightly grease a large baking sheet.

3 When the potatoes are done, drain in a colander and let cool for 10 minutes.

4 Place the potatoes on the prepared baking sheet. With the base of a cup or measuring cup, press down (a.k.a. SMASH) each potato until it's mostly flattened. Some potatoes might break apart a little, but don't worry about that.

5 Drizzle the potatoes with the oil and sprinkle with the garlic powder, salt, and pepper.

6 Roast the potatoes until they look golden brown and crispy throughout, 25 to 30 minutes. Be sure to keep a close eye on them, as they can burn.

7 Remove the potatoes from the oven and sprinkle with the dill and more salt and pepper, to taste. Serve immediately with the aioli. If you have any leftovers, they can be reheated in a toaster oven or in a frying pan.

PREP TIME:
10 minutes
COOK TIME:
30 minutes
YIELD:
8 servings

brussels sprouts slaw

8 strips bacon
2 pounds (900 g) Brussels sprouts, shredded
4 cups (600 g) thinly sliced red cabbage
1 small red onion, finely diced
⅓ cup (53 g) hemp seeds
1 batch Slaw Sauce (page 174)
Kosher salt, to taste
Black pepper, to taste

If you're a fan of slaw, you are going to be head-over-heels in love with this Brussels sprouts version. Shredded Brussels sprouts are going to increase your slaw love tenfold, and the crisp diced bacon ain't bad either. You might not use all the slaw sauce, but you're going to want to add it to all sorts of other veggies, so no worries there!

1 Line a baking sheet with parchment paper and adjust the oven rack to the middle position. Add the bacon in a single layer, place in a cold oven, and set the temperature to 375°F (190°C). The bacon will take 25 to 30 minutes to cook. Set aside to cool slightly. Once the bacon is cool enough to handle, dab it with paper towels, transfer it to a cutting board, and chop.

2 In a large bowl, add the Brussels sprouts and cabbage, tossing to combine. Add the onion, bacon, and hemp seeds and stir.

3 Add the slaw sauce, a few tablespoons at a time, until it's coated to your liking. Expect to use about ¾ cup (180 ml). Taste for salt and pepper.

NOTE:

This slaw will get even better as it sits. Stick it in the refrigerator for 2 hours or overnight if you have the time!

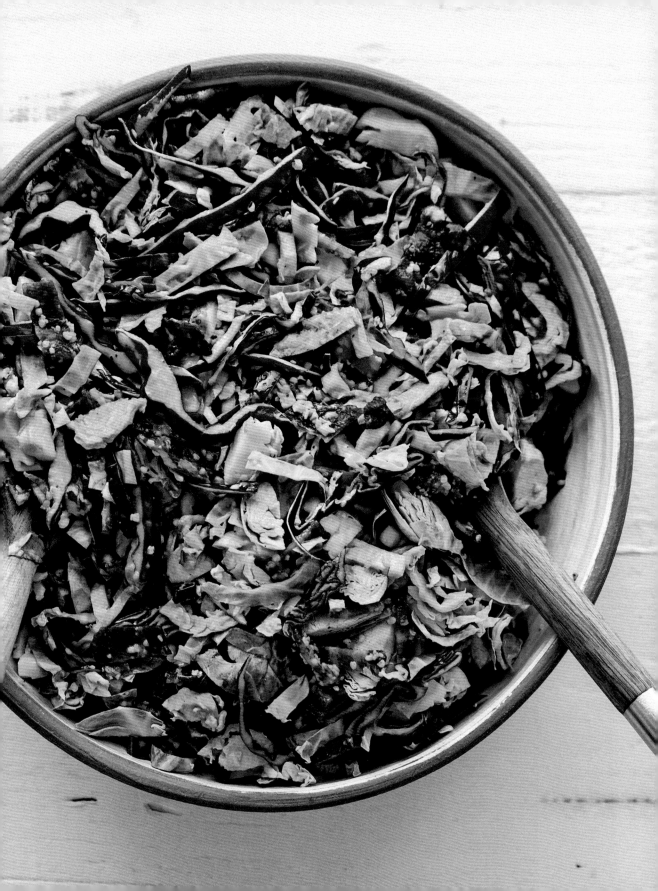

PREP TIME:
15 minutes

COOK TIME:
15 minutes

YIELD:
2 servings

crispy zucchini fritters

3 cups (450 g) lightly packed shredded zucchini

½ teaspoon kosher salt, plus more for sprinkling

½ cup (60 g) plus 2 tablespoons (15 g) cassava flour (see Note)

2 large eggs, lightly beaten

½ teaspoon garlic powder

½ teaspoon ground ginger

2 tablespoons (30 ml) ghee or coconut oil, divided

Honey Mustard Sauce (page 178), for dipping (optional)

I originally made these zucchini fritters for my daughter when she was transitioning into trying solid foods. I knew I wanted to create something that was veggie loaded but also packed with her favorite Asian spices. My girl loves ginger and garlic, and that's exactly what I put inside these fritters. They're crispy on the outside, while remaining soft and cakey on the inside. While they're fabulous on their own, my favorite way to eat them is dipped into Honey Mustard Sauce (page 178).

1   Place the zucchini in a colander in the sink and sprinkle lightly with kosher salt. Allow it to stand for 10 minutes. Rinse off the zucchini and, using your hands, squeeze out as much of the liquid as possible. You can use a towel to absorb some of the moisture. Transfer to a large bowl.

2   Add the cassava flour, eggs, garlic powder, ginger, and ½ teaspoon salt and stir until well combined. Line a big plate with paper towels and set aside.

3   Add 1 tablespoon (15 ml) of the ghee or oil to a large skillet and place over medium heat. Once hot (about 1 minute), scoop 2- or 3-tablespoon-size (30 or 45 ml) balls of the mixture into the pan, lightly pressing down to make them flatter. Space them a few inches apart and cook until brown, about 3 minutes per side. Transfer the fritters to the plate and repeat with the remaining 1 tablespoon (15 ml) oil and batter.

4   Serve with the honey mustard sauce, if using.

NOTE:

Cassava flour is gluten-free, grain-free, and nut-free and the most similar to wheat flour. Look for it at most grocery stores with the other alternative flours or purchase it online.

PREP TIME:
15 minutes

COOK TIME:
8 minutes

YIELD:
6 servings

instant pot mashed potatoes

3 pounds (1.3 kg) Yukon gold potatoes, peeled and sliced into 1- to 1½-inch (2.5 cm to 4 cm) disks

2 teaspoons (12 g) salt, divided, plus more to taste

¼ cup (60 g) grass-fed butter or ghee

½ to ¾ cup (120 to 180 ml) full-fat canned coconut milk

2½ tablespoons (37 ml) Clean Paleo Mayo (page 176)

½ teaspoon garlic powder

½ teaspoon black pepper, plus more to taste

I absolutely love this method for cooking mashed potatoes. I can get the rest of my lunch, dinner, meal prep, or whatever I need done while this beautiful side dish is cooking. The addition of mayo to the mashed potatoes gives them a texture and flavor that simply cannot be beat. You're going to love serving this to guests or having it in the refrigerator for a quick-grab meal accompaniment. De-lish!

1 Place the potatoes in the bottom of the Instant Pot.

2 Cover with 4 to 5 cups (950 ml to 1.2 L) water (depending on the size of your pot) and add 1 teaspoon (6 g) of the salt.

3 Place the lid on the Instant Pot and set the valve to Sealing.

4 Cook on Manual High pressure for 8 minutes.

5 When the timer goes off, press the Keep Warm/Cancel button and carefully release the pressure.

6 Drain the potatoes, then return them to the pot. Add the remaining 1 teaspoon (6 g) salt, along with the butter, coconut milk, mayo, garlic powder, and pepper. Mash until well combined and smooth. Taste for additional seasoning. Serve warm.

PREP TIME:
5 minutes
COOK TIME:
15 minutes
YIELD:
4 servings

GRAIN / DAIRY

truffled polenta rounds

2-ounce (56 g) chunk
   Parmesan cheese
3 tablespoons (45 ml)
   avocado oil or ghee
1 tube (14 ounces [396 g])
   polenta, cut into ¼- to
   ½-inch (6 to 13 mm) thick
   rounds
¾ teaspoon salt, divided
4 tablespoons (60 ml)
   grass-fed butter, separated
   into teaspoons
Large egg yolk, lightly beaten
Microgreens, for garnish

This is a recipe from my husband Tim's heart, and I am just a guest there sharing that space. He made this dish for me for the first time while I was pregnant, and I have requested it as often as possible since then. I love his innovation of adding extra butter to each polenta round while they are cooking—it's pure genius and it gives them so much fatty goodness and depth of flavor. These are perfect as an appetizer or as a side to any entrée.

1   Thinly slice or shave the Parmesan so you have 1½ x 1½-inch (4 x 4 cm) squares. You should have one for each round of polenta.

2   Heat a large cast-iron skillet over medium-high heat until it begins to lightly smoke, 2 minutes. Add the oil and swirl around the bottom of the pan.

3   Add the polenta rounds in a single layer, leaving space in between so they can crisp up. Sprinkle with ½ teaspoon of the salt. Cook until they begin to turn golden brown and crisp around the edges, 5 to 7 minutes. Flip over.

4   Add a square of Parmesan on top of each polenta round and cook for 3 minutes. Sprinkle with the remaining ¼ teaspoon salt and add 1 teaspoon butter per round. Cook until your desired crispness has been reached, another minute or so.

5   Transfer the rounds to plates. Drizzle with the egg yolk and top with the microgreens.

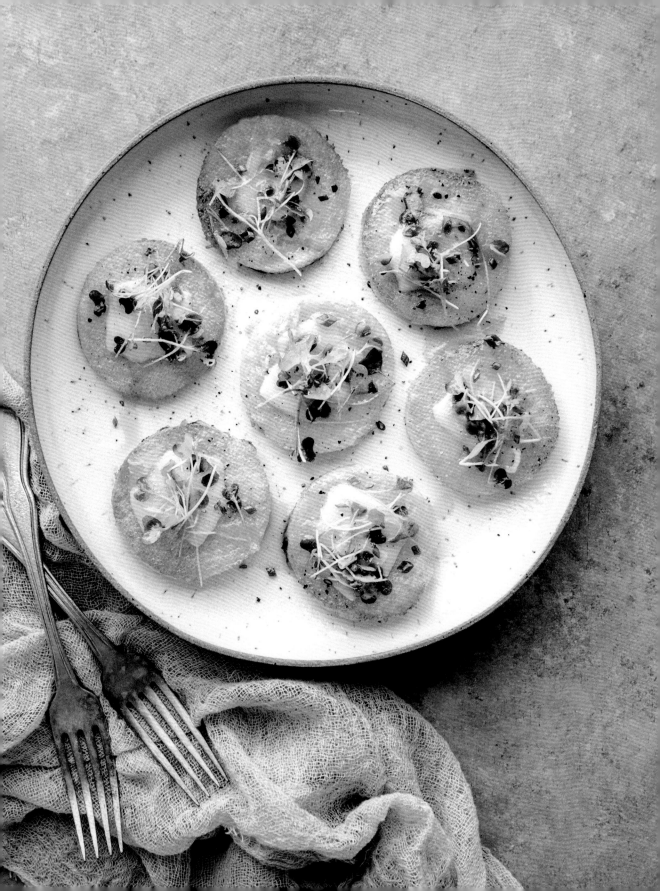

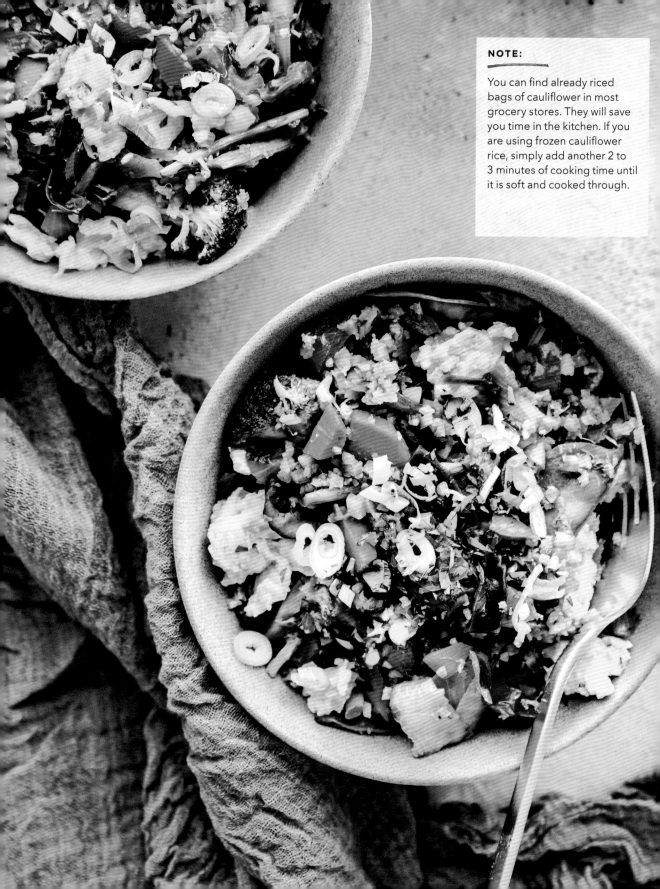

NOTE:

You can find already riced bags of cauliflower in most grocery stores. They will save you time in the kitchen. If you are using frozen cauliflower rice, simply add another 2 to 3 minutes of cooking time until it is soft and cooked through.

PREP TIME:
30 minutes

COOK TIME:
25 minutes

YIELD:
6 servings

SWEETENER

3 tablespoons (45 ml) avocado oil, divided

1 small yellow onion, diced

½ teaspoon kosher salt, plus more to taste

1 tablespoon (15 ml) toasted sesame oil

8 cloves garlic, minced

3 cups (450 g) thinly sliced red cabbage

½ bunch asparagus, ends trimmed, stalks cut into 2- to 3-inch (5 to 7.5 cm) pieces

6 ounces (169 g) cremini or baby bella mushrooms, coarsely chopped

1 red bell pepper, julienned

¼ cup (60 ml) low-sodium chicken broth

4 cups (600 g) frozen or fresh cauliflower rice (see Note)

4 to 6 large eggs

1 batch Asian Marinade/ Stir-Fry Sauce (page 175)

Black pepper, to taste

¼ cup (40 g) thinly sliced scallions, for garnish

Sesame seeds, for garnish

umami-filled cauliflower rice

I know there are a million and one recipes out there for fried cauliflower rice, but this one is going to win your vote because of the insane stir-fry sauce it's cooked with. (Make that first— it's super fast—and have all your veggies ready to go before you start cooking.) The toasted sesame oil in this dish is what really makes it taste authentic, and you won't even need to try and fool anyone because they're going to think it's over the moon. Be sure to garnish with the scallions and sesame seeds if you're wanting to keep it really, real, real. Wink.

1 Heat a very large sauté pan or wok over medium-high heat for 1 minute and add 2 tablespoons (30 ml) of the avocado oil. After another minute, add the onion and salt. Sauté until the onion appears soft and almost translucent, 4 to 5 minutes. Add the sesame oil and garlic. Sauté for another minute, until fragrant, stirring often.

2 Add the cabbage, asparagus, mushrooms, bell pepper, and broth. Give everything a nice stir and cover with a lid, stirring occasionally. Cook until the veggies are soft and nearly cooked through, 7 to 10 minutes.

3 Add the cauliflower rice. Cook until everything is fork tender and cooked through, stirring occasionally, 5 to 7 minutes more.

4 Meanwhile, in another large frying pan, turn the heat to medium. After 1 minute, add the remaining 1 tablespoon (15 ml) avocado oil. Add the eggs to the pan and cook, stirring often, until cooked through and fluffy, 3 to 4 minutes. Remove from the heat.

5 Add the stir-fry sauce to the veggies and lower the heat to medium. Cook, stirring often, until the sauce has reduced a bit, 3 to 5 minutes. Add the scrambled eggs and stir well. Taste for additional salt and add black pepper to taste. Serve right away, garnished with the scallions and sesame seeds.

PREP TIME:
15 minutes
COOK TIME:
30 minutes
YIELD:
4 servings

SWEETENER /
GRAIN / DAIRY

butternut squash–stuffed mushrooms

These stuffed portobello mushrooms make me think that I could try being a vegetarian again. Just kidding. Truly, though, these creamy and savory stuffed mushrooms are the perfect complement to your dinner. The slightly sweet squash has a hint of anise flavor, the mushrooms are spiked with garlic and thyme, and it's all topped off with some tangy sun-dried tomatoes and goat cheese. You might just want to have two and call it a meal!

SQUASH
2 cups (300 g) ½-inch (1.3 cm) diced butternut squash
1 tablespoon (15 ml) extra virgin olive oil
1 tablespoon (9 g) coconut sugar
1 heaping teaspoon (2 g) fennel seeds
Kosher salt, to taste
Black pepper, to taste

MUSHROOMS
4 cloves garlic, minced
2 tablespoons (30 ml) extra virgin olive oil
1 tablespoon (2.4 g) fresh thyme leaves, coarsely chopped
4 portobello mushroom caps, gills removed and wiped clean

FILLING
¼ cup (27.5 g) sun-dried tomatoes in oil, drained and finely chopped
¼ cup (40 g) gluten-free bread crumbs
¼ cup (37 g) crumbled goat cheese

Arugula, for serving
Fresh lemon juice, for serving
Extra virgin olive oil, for serving
Balsamic vinegar, for serving

1 Preheat the oven to 400°F (200°C). Adjust the oven rack to the middle position and line a baking sheet with parchment paper.

2 To make the squash, in a large bowl, toss together the squash, olive oil, coconut sugar, fennel seeds, and a big pinch of salt and pepper. Use your hands to toss until everything is combined. Transfer the squash to the prepared baking sheet and roast until golden, 15 to 20 minutes.

3 When finished, remove from the oven and reduce the temperature to 375°F (190°C). Line a new baking sheet with parchment paper.

4 Meanwhile, to make the mushrooms, combine the garlic, olive oil, and thyme in a small bowl. Brush the inside of each mushroom cap with this mixture.

5 To make the filling, in the same bowl, combine the sun-dried tomatoes and bread crumbs.

6 Divide the squash evenly among the mushroom caps. Top them with the tomato and bread crumb mixture. Dollop a few chunks of goat cheese on each and place on the new baking sheet.

7 Bake until the mushrooms become tender and the tops turn golden brown, 12 to 16 minutes.

8 To serve, lay each mushroom on a bed of baby arugula and drizzle with lemon juice, olive oil, and vinegar.

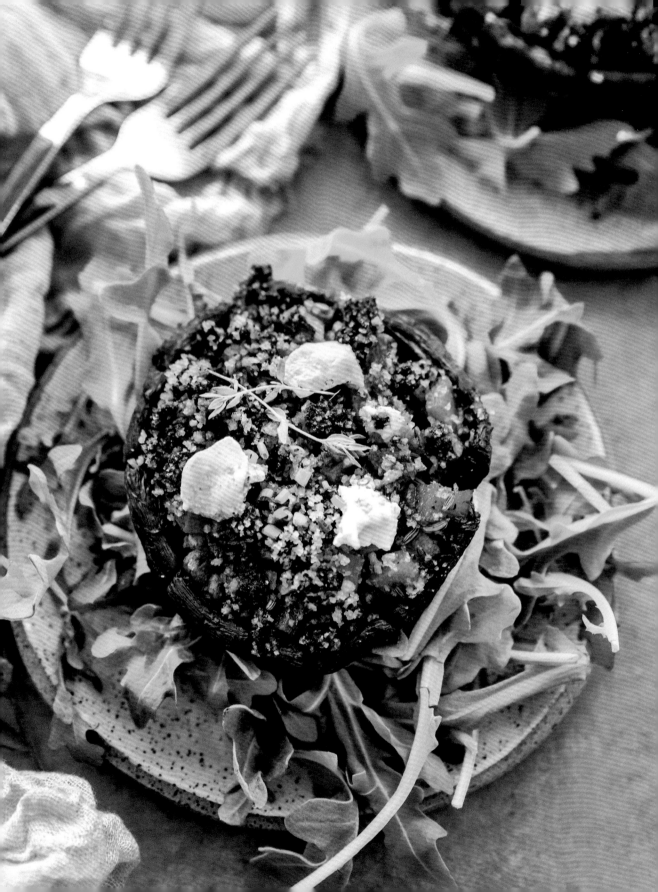

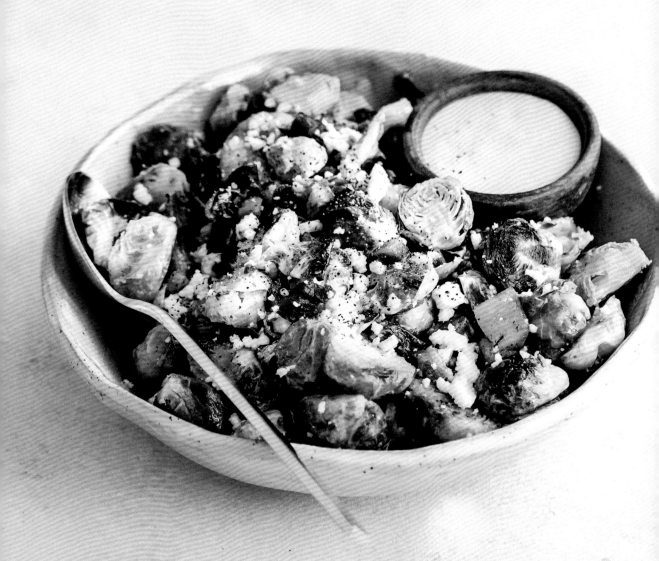

PREP TIME:
5 minutes
COOK TIME:
30 minutes
YIELD:
4 servings

DAIRY

game-changing brussels sprouts

- 4 cups (600 g) trimmed and halved Brussels sprouts
- 4 ounces (113 g) pancetta, finely diced
- 3 tablespoons (45 ml) avocado oil or extra-virgin olive oil
- 1 teaspoon (6 g) kosher salt, plus more to taste
- ¼ cup (60 g) Tomato-Garlic Aioli (page 182)
- 1 to 2 tablespoons (15 to 30 ml) filtered water
- ¼ cup (37 g) crumbled cotija cheese
- Black pepper, to taste

We've all had roasted Brussels sprouts about a million times. Though there are many ways to heighten the flavor of Brussels, I'm choosing to incorporate my favorite crumbly cheese, some smoky pancetta, and a decadent garlic-forward dipping sauce. This dish is absolutely perfect paired with a weeknight meal, or make a double or triple batch to have at your holiday spread. You really can't go wrong.

1 Preheat the oven to 400°F (200°C) and adjust the oven rack to the middle position. Line a baking sheet with parchment paper.

2 In a large bowl, combine the Brussels sprouts with the pancetta, oil, and salt. Give everything a nice toss so the sprouts are evenly coated. Transfer to the baking sheet and spread in a single layer.

3 Bake, flipping halfway through, until the pancetta is crispy and the Brussels sprouts are beginning to turn brown, 25 to 30 minutes.

4 Meanwhile, in a small bowl, mix together the aioli with the water, depending on the consistency you'd like for drizzling or dipping. Set aside.

5 Transfer the Brussels sprouts to a serving dish and top off with the cotija. Add more salt and black pepper, if desired. Serve with the tomato-garlic sauce.

PREP TIME:
5 minutes

COOK TIME:
15 minutes

YIELD:
4 servings

DAIRY

pan-roasted zucchini

3 tablespoons (45 ml) avocado oil, divided

½ yellow onion, sliced

4 medium zucchini (about 2 pounds [900 g]), cut into ½-inch (1.3 cm) rounds

1 teaspoon (6 g) kosher salt, plus more to taste

½ teaspoon garlic powder

¼ teaspoon black pepper, plus more to taste

3 tablespoons (45 ml) chicken bone broth

¼ cup (22 g) grated Parmesan cheese

There's nothing quite like a straightforward but flavorful side dish like this pan-roasted zucchini. It takes very little time to prepare and almost no time on the stove at all. You can have everything done in less than twenty minutes, and it tastes absolutely divine with the grated Parmesan on top. If you aren't into dairy, it also tastes delicious drizzled with some of my Cashew Cheese (page 174).

1 In a large skillet, heat 1½ tablespoons (22 ml) of the oil for 2 minutes over medium heat. Add the onion and cook until soft, 4 to 5 minutes.

2 Add the zucchini, salt, garlic powder, and pepper. Cook, stirring frequently, until softened, about 7 minutes. Add the broth and cook until the broth has evaporated, 2 to 3 minutes more. Add the remaining 1½ tablespoons (22 ml) oil and cook for another few minutes, until the zucchini browns on the edges.

3 Remove from the heat and sprinkle with the Parmesan. Taste and add salt and pepper as needed.

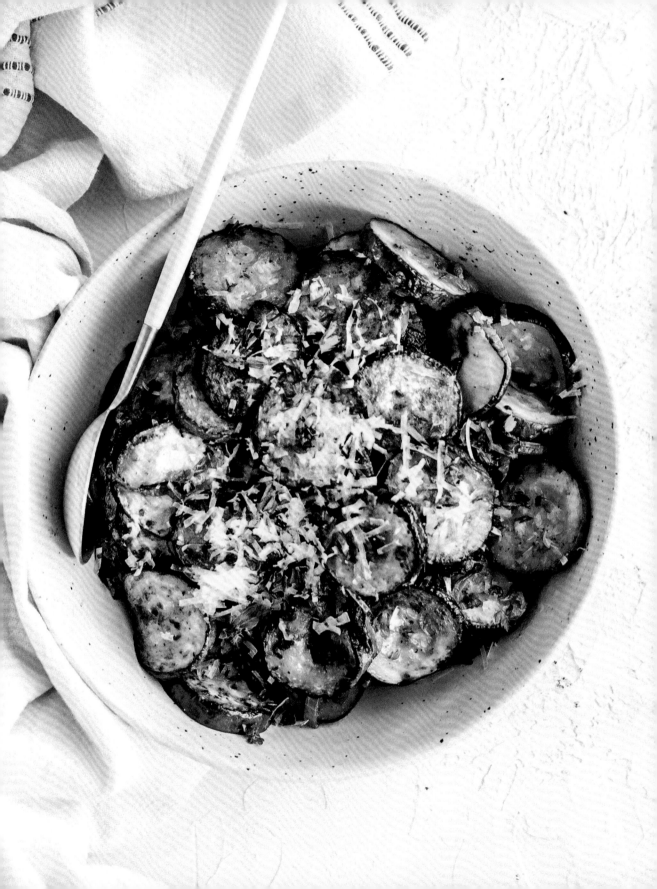

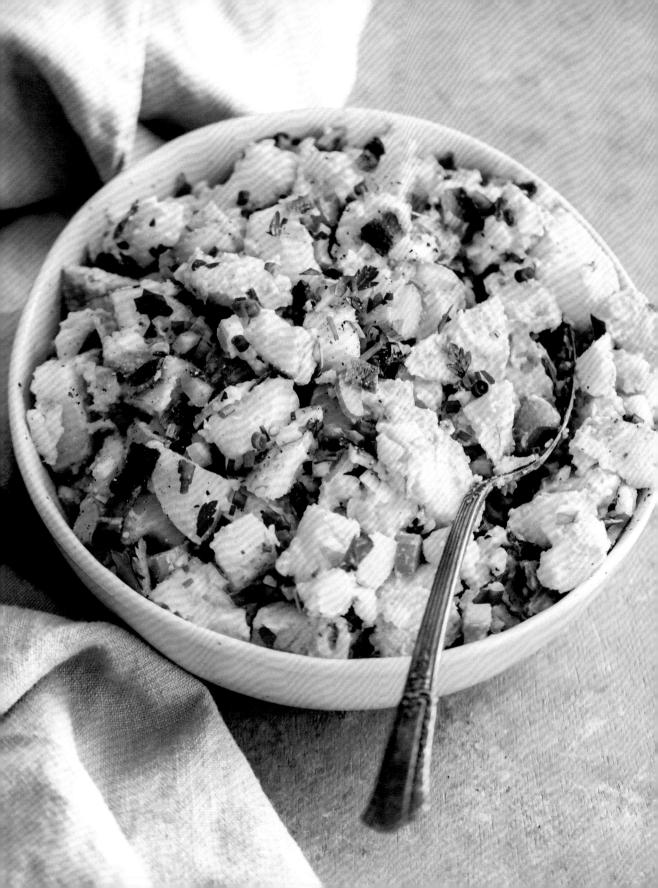

PREP TIME:
10 minutes +
cooling and
chilling time

COOK TIME:
25 minutes

YIELD:
6 to 8 servings

buffalo potato salad

3 pounds (1.3 kg) Yukon
gold potatoes, cut into
1-inch (2.5 cm) chunks

6 to 8 strips bacon, chopped

⅔ cup (160 ml) Clean Paleo
Mayo (page 176)

1 small red onion, finely
diced

½ cup (75 g) finely diced
celery

¼ cup (60 ml) hot sauce

¼ cup (5 g) fresh parsley,
coarsely chopped

2 tablespoons (30 ml) fresh
lemon juice

6 cloves garlic, minced

Handful fresh chives,
chopped, for garnish

Kosher salt, to taste

Black pepper, to taste

This creamy paleo potato salad is loaded with crunchy bacon bits, crispy red onion, and a combination of homemade paleo mayo and zesty hot sauce that'll leave you wanting more. It's the perfect side dish to serve with your favorite protein all year-round. Not to mention the fact that the sauce is so good, you are going to want to make extra and use it as a dip for anything and everything!

1 Place the potatoes in a large saucepan or Dutch oven and cover with water by 1 inch (2.5 cm). Bring to a boil over high heat. Reduce the heat to medium-low and cook until the potatoes are easily pierced with a fork and you're able to pull it out with little resistance. This should take 10 to 15 minutes.

2 Drain the water and transfer the potatoes to a large bowl. Cool in the refrigerator for 15 to 20 minutes.

3 Meanwhile, cook the bacon. Line a baking sheet with parchment paper and adjust the oven rack to the middle position. Add the bacon in a single layer, place in a cold oven, and set the temperature to 375°F (190°C). The bacon will take 25 to 30 minutes to cook. Set aside to cool slightly. Once the bacon is cool enough to handle, dab it with paper towels, transfer it to a cutting board, and chop.

4 Once the potatoes have cooled, add the bacon, mayo, onion, celery, hot sauce, parsley, lemon juice, garlic, and chives. Stir to completely coat.

5 Add salt and black pepper to taste. Refrigerate for at least an hour and serve cold.

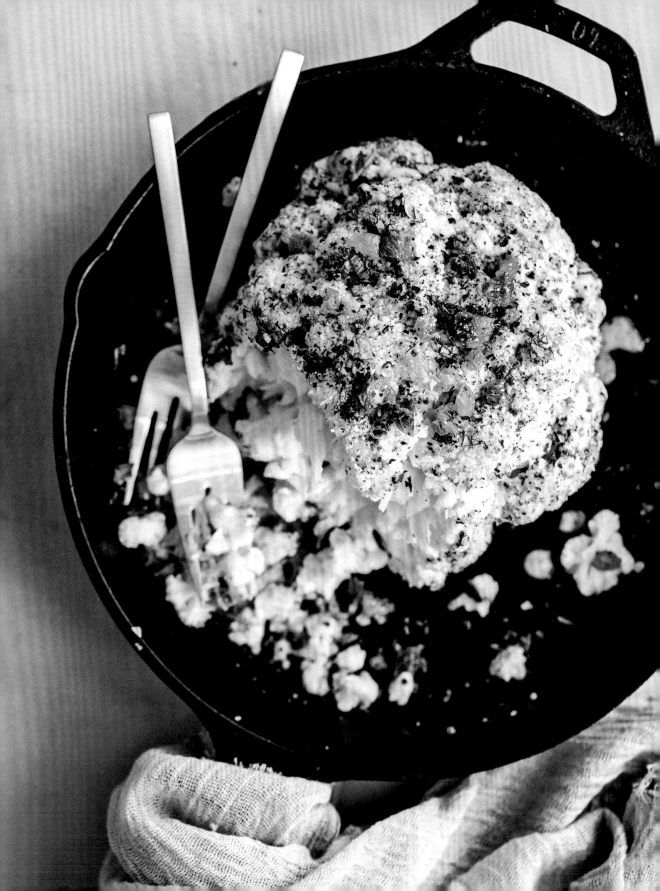

PREP TIME:
5 minutes
COOK TIME:
50 minutes
YIELD:
3 to 4 servings

DAIRY

whole roasted cauliflower with pesto, mint & raisins

1 head cauliflower, leaves removed
¼ cup (60 ml) ghee, melted
5 tablespoons (75 ml) Arugula Pesto (page 183), divided
¼ teaspoon black pepper
¼ cup (60 ml) Clean Paleo Mayo (page 176)
1 tablespoon (15 ml) filtered water
2 tablespoons (12 g) fresh mint, coarsely chopped
2 tablespoons (18 g) golden raisins, coarsely chopped
Kosher salt, to taste

If you're looking for a side dish that looks very fancy and well thought out but actually takes very little time to prepare, then look no further. This fabulous cauliflower slow cooks in the oven, lathered in arugula pesto and ghee—yum! Finished off with sweet golden raisins, fresh mint, and rich pesto aioli, this dish should be on the menu at your next dinner party.

1 Preheat the oven to 375°F (190°C) and adjust the oven rack to the middle position. Line a cast-iron pan or a baking dish with parchment paper.

2 Place the cauliflower in the pan.

3 In a small bowl, combine the ghee, 2 tablespoons (30 ml) of the pesto, and pepper until smooth throughout. Brush this mixture all over the cauliflower. Be sure to get it in all the crevices. Cover the pan with aluminum foil.

4 Bake for 30 minutes. Remove the foil and bake for an additional 15 minutes. When done, it should be easy to pierce with a fork. Set the broiler to low and broil for 5 to 7 minutes.

5 Meanwhile, combine the mayo, remaining 3 tablespoons (45 ml) pesto, and water in a bowl.

6 Remove the cauliflower from the oven and drizzle with the pesto aioli. Sprinkle with the mint, raisins, and salt before serving.

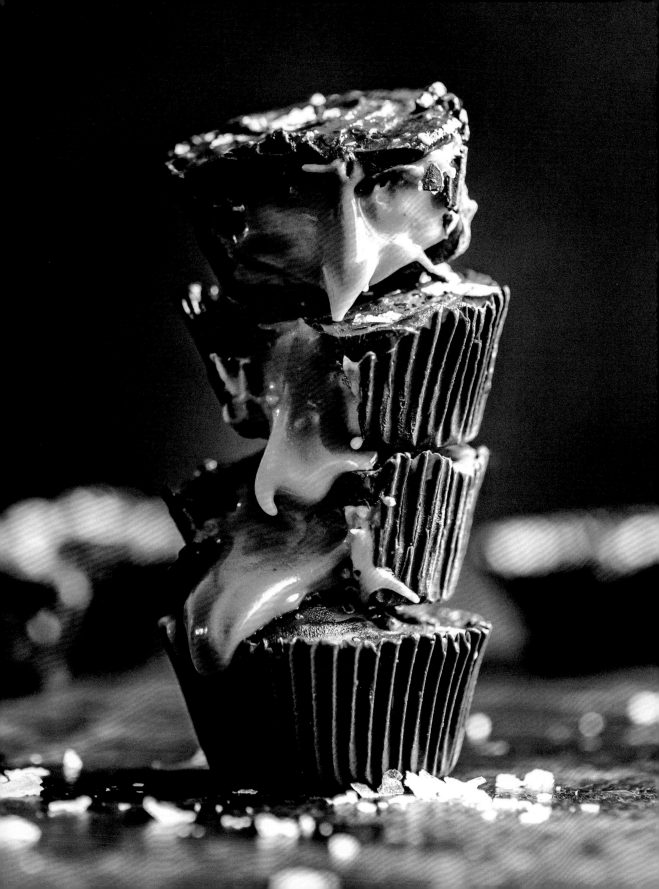

CHAPTER 8

desserts & drinks

GROWING UP IN CHICAGO, I always wanted to spend more time at my friends' houses than my own. Many of my friends' mothers were devoted bakers. I remember being so excited waking up on Saturday mornings after a slumber party to the smell of freshly made baked goods. At that time in my life, nothing was better.

Well, things really haven't changed that much. I find so much comfort and joy in baking. And following a paleo lifestyle shouldn't mean giving that up! One of my favorite desserts of all time are cookies. They're so easy to whip up to bring to a get-together or stash away in the freezer for whenever you'd like a treat. (And you can eat the cookie dough. That's a huge plus.)

Making amazing paleo-friendly desserts and drinks is really quite simple. Once you understand the basic techniques of making desserts, you can let your imagination take over. Drinks just need balance. I know I can't even start thinking about my day unless I have a morning beverage recipe on the back burner. Looking forward to that drink is a precursor to a wonderful day at my house.

In this chapter, you will find so many incredible recipes ranging from Cashew Chocolate Chip Cookies to Apple Scones with Peach Butter. There are Dark Chocolate & Caramel Cashew Butter Cups and a Bone Broth Hot Chocolate that is seriously decadent. Get ready for an incredible journey through the land of paleo desserts and drinks.

◀ Dark Chocolate & Caramel Cashew Butter Cups, page 152

PREP TIME:
5 minutes

COOK TIME:
45 minutes +
cool time

YIELD:
8 servings

SWEETENER

pumpkin bread

1 cup (150 g) raw cashews

½ cup (60 g) coconut flour

1 teaspoon (4.6 g) baking
soda

1 teaspoon (2.3 g) ground
cinnamon

½ teaspoon pumpkin pie
spice

½ teaspoon kosher salt

¼ teaspoon ground cloves

1 cup (200 g) coconut sugar

½ cup (115 g) canned
pumpkin puree

⅓ cup (80 ml) ghee or
coconut oil, melted, plus
more for the pan

¼ cup (60 ml) full-fat canned
coconut milk

1½ teaspoons (7.5 ml) pure
vanilla extract

4 large eggs

This easy paleo pumpkin bread is cashew based, which gives it a very nutty and buttery flavor. It's absolutely heavenly and extremely moist, too. Watch anyone who is not a pumpkin lover become a convert after trying this bread. My husband does not like bread, and he doesn't like pumpkin-flavored anything. Guess who ate three pieces of this in one sitting? Yep.

1 Preheat the oven to 325°F (170°C). Adjust the oven rack to the middle position. Lightly coat the bottom and sides of a 9 x 5-inch (23 x 12.5 cm) loaf pan with extra ghee or oil. Cut a piece of parchment paper to fit the length of the bottom of the pan and leave some extra parchment hanging over the sides so you can easily lift out the loaf.

2 To make the cashew flour, pulse the cashews in a food processor, a few seconds at a time, until they resemble a coarse meal. You don't want any visible chunks of cashews. This should take about 1 minute.

3 Add the coconut flour, baking soda, cinnamon, pumpkin pie spice, salt, and cloves. Pulse several times, until well mixed. Add the coconut sugar, pumpkin, ghee or oil, coconut milk, vanilla, and eggs. Process for another 30 to 45 seconds, until well combined. Scrape down the sides if necessary during this process to make sure everything has been well incorporated.

4 Using a spatula, transfer the pumpkin mixture to the prepared loaf pan. Tap it on the counter multiple times to release any air bubbles and smooth over the top with an offset spatula. Bake until a toothpick inserted into the center comes out clean, 40 to 45 minutes. A few crumbs are okay, but you don't want any raw batter.

5 Let the bread cool in the pan for 30 minutes before using a knife to loosen it around the edges and transferring it to a wire rack to cool completely. Slice and serve.

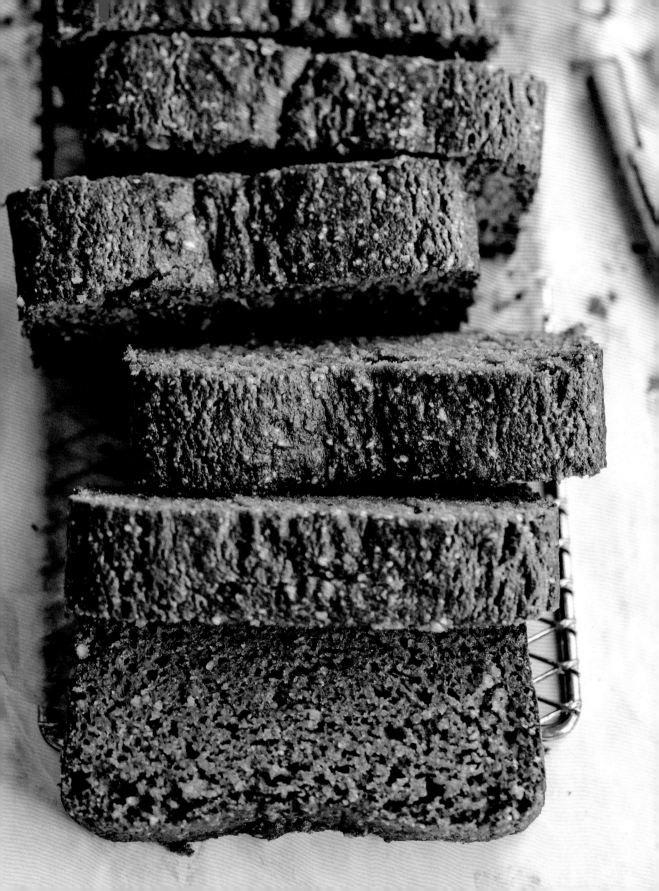

PREP TIME:
10 minutes +
freeze time

COOK TIME:
5 minutes

YIELD:
24 cups

SWEETENER

2½ cups (450 g) dark
chocolate chunks, divided
½ cup (125 g) creamy cashew
butter or peanut butter
⅓ cup (50 g) macadamia
nuts, crushed
1 batch Easy Vegan Caramel
Sauce (page 153, see Note)
Flaky sea salt, for topping

NOTE:

If you don't have the
caramel sauce already
made, get it going first;
the candies can hang out
in the freezer in step 3
until it's ready.

dark chocolate & caramel cashew butter cups

These creamy dark chocolate cups are the best dang treat ever. They are oozing with homemade caramel sauce, creamy cashew butter, and crushed macadamia nuts. This is my go-to recipe if I have a friend or family member's birthday coming up. They freeze extremely well and make the best gift ever!

1 Line a mini cupcake pan with 24 parchment liners.

2 Melt 1¼ cups (225 g) of the chocolate chunks. You can either use a double boiler or heat them in a bowl in the microwave for 45 seconds at a time, stirring after each interval.

3 Drop 1 teaspoon (5 ml) of the melted chocolate into each liner. Now, smooth the chocolate up the sides of the liner with the back of a small spoon. Place the tray in the freezer for about 10 minutes to set.

4 Take out the tray and add 1 teaspoon (5 g) of cashew butter to each chocolate cup. Return the tray to the freezer for another 10 minutes.

5 Take the tray out of the freezer and divide the macadamia nuts among the cups. Top each chocolate cup with 2 teaspoons (10 ml) of caramel. Place back in the freezer.

6 Melt the remaining 1¼ cups (225 g) chocolate chunks and cover the candy with it. Sprinkle the tops with some sea salt. Let them harden in the freezer for 1 hour, then store in an airtight container in the refrigerator for up to 1 week or in the freezer for up to 2 months.

PREP TIME:
5 minutes

COOK TIME:
40 minutes

YIELD:
about 1 cup
(240 ml)

SWEETENER

easy vegan caramel sauce

1 can (13.5 ounces [382 g]) full-fat coconut milk
½ cup (100 g) coconut sugar
2 tablespoons (30 ml) pure maple syrup
¼ teaspoon kosher salt
1½ teaspoons (7.5 ml) coconut oil
1½ teaspoons (7.5 ml) pure vanilla extract

The best vegan caramel sauce recipe is on deck, made with creamy coconut milk, pure maple syrup and other natural, real-food ingredients. It takes very little effort to make on the stove and is so lovely as a topping for ice cream, a dip for apples, or just eaten straight with a spoon. It's the secret ingredient in my Dark Chocolate & Caramel Cashew Butter Cups (page 152), and I can't wait you for to try it!

1   In a medium saucepan, combine the coconut milk, coconut sugar, maple syrup, and salt over medium-high heat.

2   Bring the mixture to a boil, whisking constantly. Turn the heat down to a simmer. Cook for 30 to 40 minutes, stirring occasionally and scraping browned bits from the bottom until the mixture has thickened. This will happen during the last few minutes.

3   Remove from the heat and stir in the coconut oil and vanilla. Let the mixture cool for a few minutes before enjoying.

4   Store in an airtight container in the refrigerator for up to 10 days. This will keep in the freezer for up to 2 months as well.

PREP TIME:
5 minutes

COOK TIME:
20 minutes +
cool time

YIELD:
12 or 16 squares

SWEETENER

five-minute chocolate chip blondies

1 cup (150 g) raw cashews
1 teaspoon (4.6 g) baking
  soda
¼ teaspoon kosher salt
½ cup (125 g) cashew butter
¼ cup (60 ml) ghee or
  coconut oil, plus more for
  the pan
¾ cup (150 g) coconut sugar
1 large egg
1 tablespoon (15 ml) pure
  vanilla extract
4 ounces (113 g) dark
  chocolate, chopped into
  chunks
Flaky sea salt, for topping

There's a new chocolate chip recipe in town, and it takes just five minutes to prep! These blondies are going to change your life. You can throw all the ingredients into the food processor and have the best grain-free, dairy-free, and paleo dessert ready in no time. Topped off with dark chocolate chunks and flaky sea salt, they make for an absolutely irresistible treat!

1 Preheat the oven to 350°F (180°C). Lightly coat an 8 x 8-inch (20.5 x 20.5 cm) baking pan with extra ghee or oil and line with parchment paper (see Note).

2 Pulse the cashews in a food processor for a few seconds at a time until they resemble a coarse meal. Make sure there are no visible chunks of cashews. This should take about 1 minute. Be sure not to turn this cashew flour into cashew butter. Watch the texture closely. Add the baking soda and kosher salt and pulse a couple of times to distribute.

3 Add the cashew butter, ghee or oil, coconut sugar, egg, and vanilla and pulse until smooth. Pulse in the chocolate chunks, just enough to distribute but not enough to break down the chocolate.

4 Use an offset spatula to spread the batter evenly in the prepared baking pan.

5 Bake until it is lightly browned around the edges and a toothpick inserted into the center comes out clean, 18 to 22 minutes.

6 Let cool in the pan completely (at least 30 minutes) before using the parchment wings to lift the blondies out of the pan. Cut into 12 or 16 squares and sprinkle with the sea salt.

7 Store in the refrigerator in an airtight container for up to 4 days. These also taste fabulous right out of the refrigerator or freezer!

NOTE:

When you measure out the parchment paper, make sure it's long enough to line the entire bottom of the pan and up both sides with a few inches (cm) of overhang on either side.

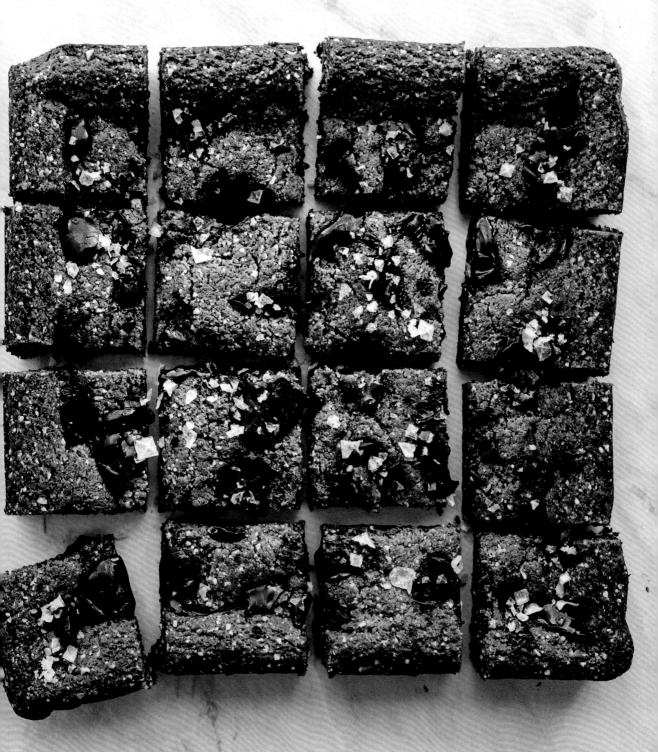

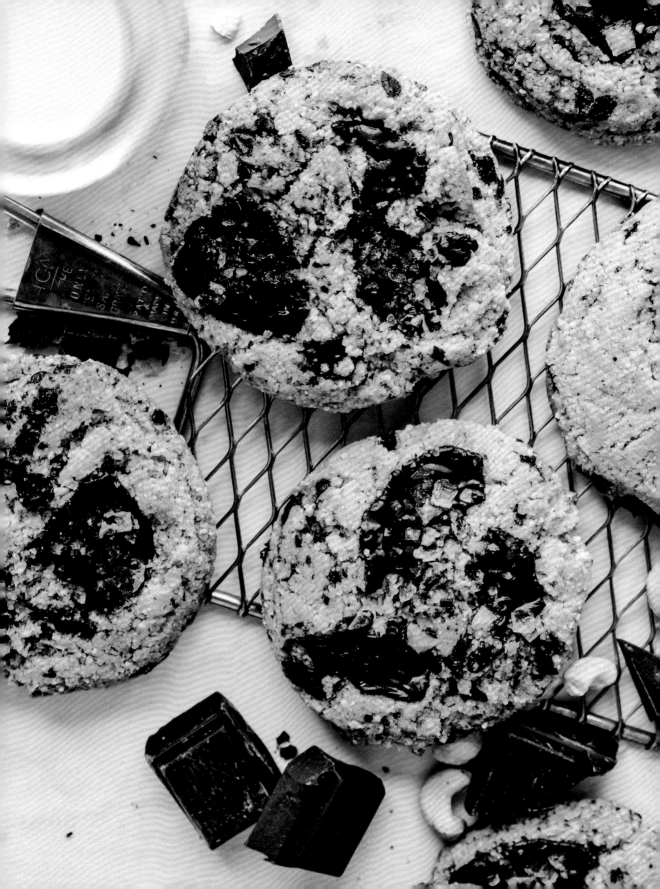

PREP TIME:
30 minutes

COOK TIME:
15 minutes +
cool time

YIELD:
10 to 12 cookies

SWEETENER

2 cups (300 g) raw cashews

¼ cup (30 g) coconut flour

2 tablespoons (18.7 g)
grass-fed gelatin
(see Note)

2 tablespoons (18 g)
coconut sugar

1½ teaspoons (7 g)
baking soda

½ teaspoon kosher salt

½ cup (120 ml) ghee,
melted

¼ cup (60 ml) pure
maple syrup

1½ teaspoons (7.5 ml)
pure vanilla extract

⅔ cup (100 g) dark
chocolate chunks
(72% to 85% cacao)

Flaky sea salt, for topping
(optional)

NOTE:

You can omit the gelatin
and replace it with 1 large
egg. However, I highly
recommend using gelatin as
it provides the best texture.

cashew chocolate chip cookies

This recipe puts a wild spin on the traditional chocolate chip cookie. You'll go nuts over these cashew-based mounds of chocolaty goodness. They are crunchy, chewy, and soft—thanks to the gelatin. Be sure to top them with flaky sea salt, if that's your jam. Just delicious!

1 Pulse the cashews in a food processor for a few seconds at a time until they resemble a coarse meal. Make sure there are no visible chunks of cashews. This should take about 1 minute. Be sure not to turn this cashew flour into cashew butter. Watch the texture closely.

2 Add the coconut flour, gelatin, coconut sugar, baking soda, and kosher salt and pulse a few more times, until everything has been well incorporated.

3 Add the ghee, maple syrup, and vanilla and give it a few more pulses. Transfer to a bowl and stir in the chocolate chunks.

4 Set the bowl in the refrigerator for 20 minutes and preheat the oven to 350°F (180°C). Place the rack in the middle of the oven and line a baking sheet with parchment paper.

5 Use a cookie scoop to form cookies and place them 2 inches (5 cm) apart on the prepared baking sheet. I use a medium-size cookie scoop. If you use a smaller one, be sure to keep an eye on the oven. Press down very lightly to flatten to the thickness you prefer (the cookies won't spread much).

6 Sprinkle some dark chocolate chunks on top if you'd like. Bake for 15 minutes, or until they start turning golden brown around the edges.

7 Leave the cookies on the baking sheet to cool completely, at least 30 minutes. Top off with flaky sea salt, if desired, before devouring.

8 These cookies will keep for up to 1 month in the freezer or 3 days in an airtight container in the refrigerator.

PREP TIME:
15 minutes +
cashew soak
and freeze time

COOK TIME:
N/A

YIELD:
12 to 16 servings

SWEETENER

build-your-own vegan & paleo cheesecake

BASE
2 cups (300 g) raw cashews
⅔ cup (160 ml) full-fat canned
    coconut milk
⅓ cup (80 ml) pure maple syrup
¼ cup (60 ml) coconut oil,
    melted and cooled to room
    temperature
2½ tablespoons (37 ml) fresh
    lemon juice
2 teaspoons (10 ml) pure
    vanilla extract

CRUST
⅔ cup (100 g) pecans or
    macadamia nuts
⅓ cup (50 g) walnuts
6 to 8 Medjool dates, pitted
¼ cup (19 g) unsweetened
    coconut flakes
Pinch of salt

TOPPING
1 cup (150 g) raspberries,
    strawberries, or blueberries
2 to 3 tablespoons (30 to 45 ml)
    pure maple syrup (see Note)

What's so awesome about this vegan paleo cheesecake recipe is that you can get creative with your crust and topping. Feel free to use whatever kind of nuts and berries you'd like, or even experiment with other fruits, adjusting the sweetener amount accordingly. The base is so easy to whip up, and you will seriously stun whoever tries it when you tell them it doesn't actually have any cream cheese in it. It's creamy and perfectly balanced—a refreshing and fabulous treat.

1   To make the base, put the cashews in a bowl and cover with boiling water. Let sit, uncovered, for 1½ hours. Rinse with cold water and drain thoroughly.

2   Meanwhile, get started on the crust. Line the bottom of a 6- or 7-inch (15 or 18 cm) springform pan with a parchment paper circle and lightly oil the sides of the pan.

3   Combine the pecans or macadamia nuts and walnuts in a food processor and pulse until coarse. Add the 6 dates, coconut flakes, and salt and pulse several times until it starts clumping together. When you press some of the mixture with your fingertips against the side of the food processor bowl, it should stick together; if it doesn't, add another 1 or 2 dates and process again.

4   Transfer the crust mixture to the pan. Press down with your fingers to pack it evenly into the bottom of the pan. If it starts to get sticky, lightly wet your fingers with warm water. Set aside.

5   Now continue with the base. Add the drained cashews, coconut milk, maple syrup, coconut oil, lemon juice, and vanilla to the cleaned bowl of your food processor or to the pitcher of a high-speed blender. Process or blend until creamy and smooth throughout, scraping down the sides as needed.

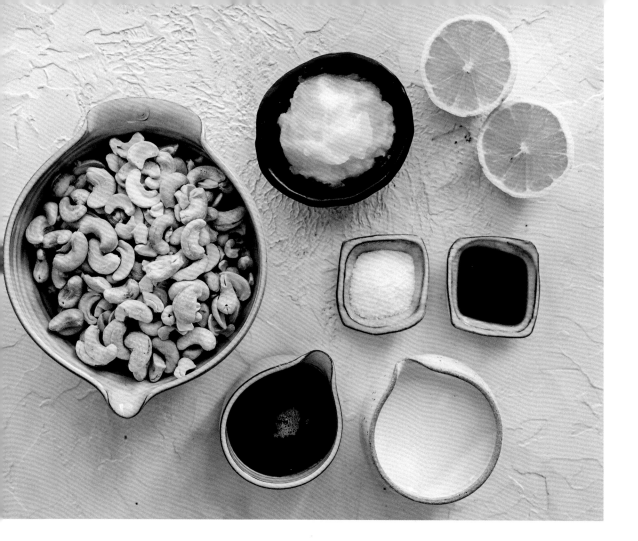

6 Pour the mixture over the crust. Tap the pan on the counter a couple
   of times to release any air bubbles that may have formed. Set aside.

7 To make the topping, combine the berries and syrup in the bowl of a
   food processor and pulse until pulverized. Spread the mixture on top
   of the filling.

8 Cover lightly with plastic wrap and transfer to the freezer for 4 to
   6 hours or overnight.

9 When ready to serve, pull the cheesecake from the fridge and allow
   it to sit at room temperature for about 15 minutes before unmolding,
   slicing, and serving.

10 Store leftovers in the freezer for up to 2 weeks.

PREP TIME:
10 minutes

COOK TIME:
32 minutes

YIELD:
8 scones

SWEETENER / DAIRY

apple scones with peach butter

SCONES
1½ cups (225 g) raw cashews
¼ cup (30 g) arrowroot flour
1 teaspoon (4.6 g) baking powder
¼ teaspoon kosher salt
¼ cup (60 ml) coconut oil, melted and cooled to room temperature
2½ tablespoons (37 ml) pure maple syrup
1½ teaspoons (7.5 ml) pure vanilla extract
1 large egg
⅔ cup (100 g) peeled and finely diced tart apple (such as Granny Smith)
⅔ cup (100 g) peeled and finely diced sweet apple (see Note)
Nondairy milk, for brushing
Cane sugar, for sprinkling

PEACH BUTTER
½ cup (120 g) grass-fed butter, at room temperature
2 tablespoons (18 g) coconut sugar
Pinch of sea salt
½ cup (75 g) peeled and diced peaches (see Note)

There is something about baking scones that leaves me feeling all warm and fuzzy inside. Maybe it's because I associate scone eating with being quite proper, and who doesn't want to feel proper? These scones come out very moist and structured, yet they are still soft and light with a crisp outside. The bits of tart and sweet apple on the inside complement the spreadable peach butter. Make these and invite all your fancy friends over for scones and tea.

1   Preheat the oven to 350°F (180°C) and adjust the oven rack to the middle position. Line an 8-inch (20 cm) cast-iron pan with parchment paper.

2   To make the scones, in the bowl of a food processor, make the cashew flour by pulsing the cashews, a few seconds at a time, until they resemble a coarse meal. There should be no visible chunks of cashews. This should take about 1 minute. Add the arrowroot flour, baking powder, and salt. Pulse a few more times until well combined.

3   In a large bowl, whisk together the coconut oil, maple syrup, vanilla, and egg. Stir the dry ingredients into the wet until well incorporated. Stir in the apples.

4   Pour the mixture into the prepared pan. Brush with milk and sprinkle with cane sugar. Bake until the edges look golden brown and a toothpick inserted into the center comes out clean, 28 to 32 minutes. Let cool in the pan for at least 10 to 15 minutes before removing from the pan and cutting into 8 scones.

5   Meanwhile, prepare the peach butter. In the bowl of a stand mixer fitted with the paddle attachment or in a large bowl using a hand mixer, whip the butter on medium-low speed until fluffy, about 1 minute. Slowly add the coconut sugar and sea salt. Continue whipping for another minute, then stir in the diced peaches. Serve on top of the warm scones.

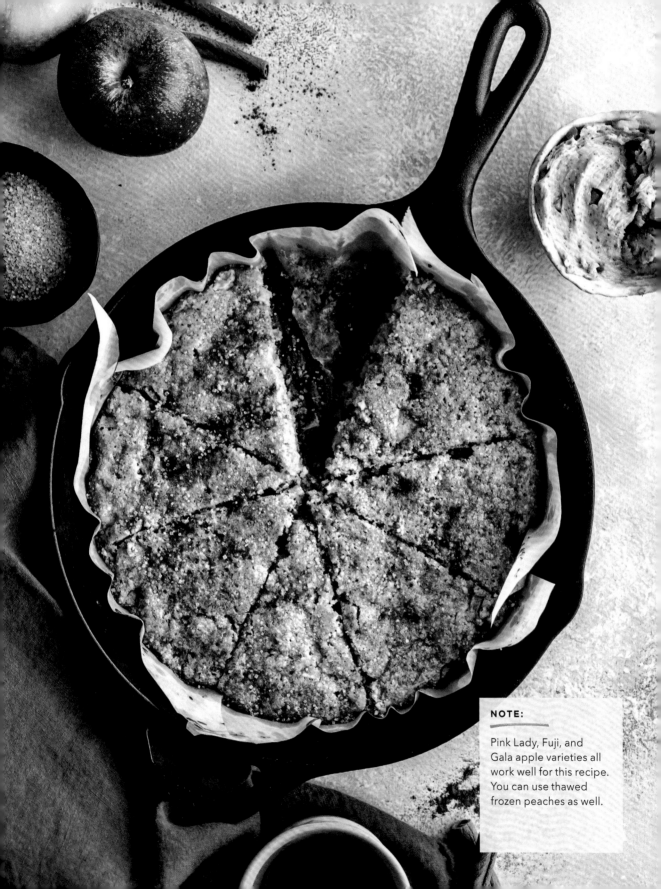

NOTE:

Pink Lady, Fuji, and Gala apple varieties all work well for this recipe. You can use thawed frozen peaches as well.

PREP TIME:
5 minutes

COOK TIME:
N/A

YIELD:
4 servings

SWEETENER

avocado chocolate pudding

⅔ cup (130 g) coconut sugar

2 avocados, peeled and pitted

⅔ cup (160 ml) full-fat canned coconut milk

½ cup (50 g) cacao powder

1 teaspoon (5 ml) pure vanilla extract

¼ teaspoon sea salt

2 to 3 tablespoons (30 to 45 ml) avocado oil or coconut oil, melted

Are you wanting to try a decadent and delicious treat that's chock-full of nourishing fats? I bet you are. This chocolate pudding is sweetened with coconut sugar and loaded with real cacao powder, sea salt, and yes, real avocados (but you would never know it!). It's such a nice indulgence that will keep you full with all those healthy fats. I like to enjoy it alongside breakfast—or as a dessert, of course. It's great plain, but you can dress it up with cacao nibs, unsweetened coconut flakes, fresh mint, etc.

1 In a food processor, pulse the coconut sugar for a few seconds. Add the avocados, coconut milk, cacao, vanilla, and salt. Process for about 1 minute until smooth, creamy, and thick throughout.

2 Turn the food processor on low and open the shoot. Slowly drizzle in the oil, 1 tablespoon (15 ml) at a time, until the mixture reaches your desired consistency. I like to use 2½ to 3 tablespoons (37 to 45 ml).

3 Store in an airtight container in the refrigerator for up to 5 days.

PREP TIME:
5 minutes +
freeze time

COOK TIME:
5 minutes

YIELD:
36 squares

SWEETENER

- 1½ cups (375 g) creamy cashew butter (see Notes)
- 1 cup (240 ml) coconut oil
- ½ cup (120 ml) pure maple syrup
- ¼ teaspoon salt
- 4 scoops collagen peptides
- 2 tablespoons (10 g) cacao powder
- 1½ tablespoons (7.5 g) Chaga powder (see Notes)
- 1½ teaspoons (7.5 g) Reishi powder (see Notes)
- 1½ teaspoons (7.5 g) mesquite powder
- ¼ cup (44 g) dark chocolate chips
- 1 teaspoon (5 ml) coconut oil

NOTES:

Almond butter will work fine, but I prefer the taste of this fudge with cashew!

You can find Chaga and Reishi in most health food stores, usually in the supplements section. They may also be with the tea and/or coffee. Mesquite powder can usually be found amongst cacao powders and online.

nut butter fudge with reishi & chaga

This creamy nut butter fudge is the best treat ever—it's both extremely decadent and refreshing because it's eaten right from the freezer. Adding Reishi and Chaga mushroom powders, cacao, and mesquite provides lovely antioxidants, while the nuts and collagen serve up a healthy dose of fat and protein. This fudge is perfect as a snack or dessert!

1 In a medium saucepan, combine the cashew butter, coconut oil, maple syrup, and salt over very low heat. Whisk until thoroughly combined and creamy, 4 minutes. Remove from the heat and whisk in the collagen, cacao, Chaga, Reishi, and mesquite.

2 Meanwhile, using a double boiler or a microwave, melt the dark chocolate chips and coconut oil over low heat or in 30-second increments, stirring in between. Set aside.

3 Line an 8 x 8-inch (20.5 x 20.5 cm) baking pan with parchment paper. Pour the fudge into the pan and tap it on the counter so it spreads evenly across the bottom.

4 Drizzle the chocolate over the fudge and use a butter knife or toothpick to swirl it.

5 Transfer the fudge to the freezer to set for at least 4 hours. When ready to serve, cut it into 36 squares. Be sure to use a hot knife to make it easier (run the knife under hot water for several seconds and dry it with a towel between slicing).

6 Store the fudge in an airtight container in the freezer for up to 1 month.

PREP TIME:
15 minutes
COOK TIME:
30 minutes
YIELD:
12 servings

SWEETENER

NUT LAYER
½ cup (75 g) pecans
½ cup (75 g) walnuts
¼ cup (60 g) grass-fed butter,
  ghee, or coconut oil, plus
  more for the pan
2 tablespoons (30 ml) pure
  maple syrup
Pinch of kosher salt

CAKE
¾ cup (90 g) coconut flour
¾ cup (90 g) arrowroot flour
2 teaspoons (7 g) baking
  powder
½ teaspoon kosher salt
4 large eggs, at room
  temperature
½ cup (120 ml) full-fat canned
  coconut milk
⅓ cup (80 ml) pure maple
  syrup
¼ cup (60 ml) ghee or
  coconut oil, melted
½ teaspoon pure vanilla
  extract

TOPPING
½ cup (75 g) pecans or
  walnuts
4 pitted dates
1 tablespoon (7 g) ground
  cinnamon
1 teaspoon (5 ml) coconut oil
Pinch of kosher salt

cinnamon crumb coffee cake

The only fond memory I have from my time working at a big coffee chain is their addictive cinnamon crumb coffee cake. What sends my version over the edge is the top layer. The crunchy combination of nuts and dates prepares you for what's to come: soft, pillowy layers of cinnamon cake.

1 Preheat the oven to 350°F (180°C) and adjust the oven rack to the middle position. Lightly grease an 8 x 8-inch (20.5 x 20.5 cm) baking dish with ghee or coconut oil.

2 To make the nut layer, combine the pecans, walnuts, butter, syrup, and salt in a food processor. Pulse until the mixture resembles a thick paste. Set aside.

3 To make the cake, in a medium bowl, sift together the coconut flour, arrowroot flour, baking powder, and salt.

4 In a separate medium bowl, whisk together the eggs, coconut milk, maple syrup, ghee or oil, and vanilla. Add to the dry mixture, mixing until smooth. The batter will be pretty thick, and that is fine.

5 Pour half the cake batter into the prepared baking dish.

6 Spread half of the nut layer on top of the cake. Pour on the rest of the cake batter, then spread the remaining nut mixture on top.

7 Bake until a toothpick inserted into the center comes out clean, 28 to 34 minutes. While the cake is in the oven, rinse and dry the food processor.

8 To make the topping, add the pecans or walnuts, dates, cinnamon, oil, and salt to the food processor. Pulse until crumbly.

9 After removing the cake from the oven, sprinkle on the topping and press it lightly into the cake. Allow to cool for at least 30 minutes.

10 Store in an airtight container in the refrigerator for up to 4 days. Eat it at room temperature or lightly toast it in the toaster oven.

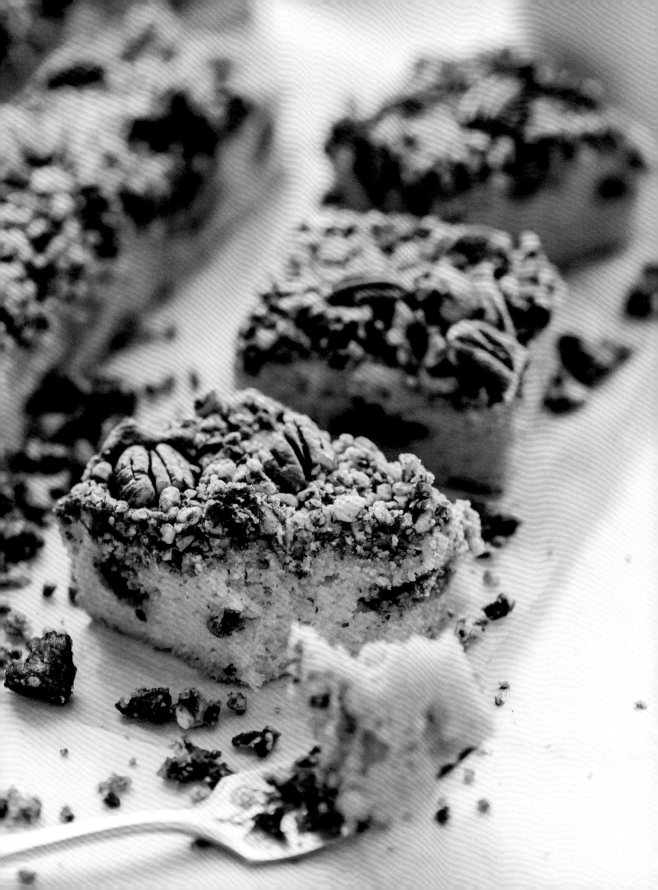

PREP TIME:
20 minutes +
cashew soak
and freeze time

COOK TIME:
N/A

YIELD:
12 to 16 bars

SWEETENER

chocolate chip cookie dough cheesecake bars

CASHEW CHEESECAKE
1½ cups (225 g) raw cashews
½ cup (120 ml) full-fat canned coconut milk
¼ cup (60 ml) pure maple syrup
3 tablespoons (45 ml) coconut oil, melted and cooled to room temperature
1½ teaspoons (7.5 ml) fresh lemon juice
1½ teaspoons (7.5 ml) pure vanilla extract

COOKIE DOUGH
2 cups (300 g) raw cashews
¼ cup (30 g) coconut flour
2 tablespoons (18.7 g) grass-fed gelatin
2 tablespoons (18 g) coconut sugar
1½ teaspoons (7 g) baking soda
½ teaspoon kosher salt
½ cup (120 ml) ghee or grass-fed butter, melted
¼ cup (60 ml) pure maple syrup
1½ teaspoons (7.5 ml) pure vanilla extract
⅔ cup plus ¼ cup (116 g plus 44 g) dark chocolate chunks, divided
1 teaspoon (5 ml) coconut oil

What if you took the best of two dessert worlds and morphed them into one? Well, then you'd have a chocolate chip cookie dough cheesecake, and it would be out-of-this-world good. I've revised my cheesecake recipe from page 158 a bit and have sandwiched that filling in between my chocolate chip cookie dough. I cannot wait for you to try this serious decadence. The filling is refreshing, while the cookie outside is mouthwateringly delicious. It's a dangerous combo.

1   Line a 9 x 5-inch (23 x 13 cm) loaf pan with parchment paper.

2   To make the cheesecake, put 1½ cups (225 g) cashews in a bowl and cover them with boiling water. Let sit, uncovered, for 1½ hours. Rinse with cold water and drain thoroughly. Set aside.

3   Meanwhile, make the cookie dough. To make the cashew flour, pulse 2 cups (300 g) raw cashews in a food processor or high-speed blender, a few seconds at a time, until they resemble a coarse meal. There should not be any visible chunks of cashews. This should take about 1 minute. Be sure not to turn the cashew flour into cashew butter. Watch the texture closely.

4   Add the coconut flour, gelatin, coconut sugar, baking soda, and salt to the food processor and pulse a few more times, until everything has been well incorporated.

5   Add the ghee, maple syrup, and vanilla and give it a few more pulses until the mixture comes together. Pulse in ⅔ cup (116 g) of the chocolate chunks, but do not process the chunks too much.

6 Transfer three-quarters of the cookie dough to the prepared loaf pan and press evenly into the bottom using wet fingers and an offset spatula. Set aside.

7 Now finish the cheesecake. Add the drained cashews to the clean bowl of your food processor or clean pitcher of a high-speed blender, along with the coconut milk, maple syrup, coconut oil, lemon juice, and vanilla. Process or blend until creamy and smooth throughout, scraping down the sides as needed.

8 Spread the cheesecake layer on top of the cookie dough crust and tap the pan on the counter multiple times to release any air bubbles. Put in the freezer to set for 2 hours.

9 Using a double boiler or a glass bowl in the microwave, melt the remaining ¼ cup (44 g) chocolate chunks with the coconut oil in 30-second increments, stirring in between. Set aside.

10 Crumble the remaining cookie dough and gently press it into the cheesecake mixture. Drizzle with the melted chocolate. Return the pan to the freezer for 2 more hours or overnight.

11 When ready to serve, pull the pan out of the freezer and let it sit at room temperature for about 30 minutes. Carefully transfer to a cutting board, and slice into 12 to 16 bars with a very sharp, wet knife.

12 Store in an airtight container in the freezer for up to 1 month. They can be stored in the refrigerator for up to 2 hours before serving.

PREP TIME:
2 to 3 minutes
COOK TIME:
N/A
YIELD:
1 serving

the best matcha latte

- 1 heaping teaspoon (2 g) Matcha powder (see Notes)
- 1½ cups (360 g) filtered water, heated to 170°F (77°C)
- 2 scoops collagen peptides (optional, see Notes)
- 1 tablespoon (15 ml) ghee, coconut butter, or MCT oil (see Notes)
- ½ teaspoon Maca powder (optional)
- ¼ teaspoon ground cinnamon (optional)

I've got all the makings for a wonderful Matcha latte recipe for you, and it's really so easy to do it yourself at home. It is made with just a few simple ingredients, but I've provided optional add-ins to really take it to the next level if you'd like. The Maca is great for hormonal health and energy, and the collagen peptides add creaminess, protein, and amino acids. This Matcha is sugar-free, dairy-free, and can be made vegan, too!

1 Using a sifter, add the Matcha powder to a 16-ounce (475 ml) mug. Using a Matcha whisk, combine with 2 tablespoons (30 ml) of 170°F (77°C) water, swirling to make figure-eight formations. Once no clumps remain, continue.

2 Transfer the mixture to the pitcher of a high-speed blender along with the remaining 1 cup and 6 tablespoons (330 ml) water, collagen (if using), ghee, Maca (if using), and cinnamon (if using). Blend on high speed for 1 minute, until creamy and frothy throughout. Serve right away.

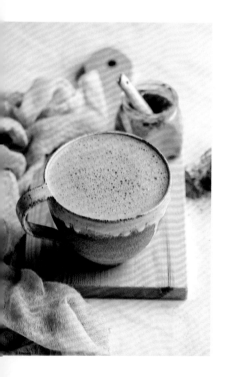

NOTES:

I recommend using a ceremonial-grade Matcha. Its flavor is above the rest and it is meant for drinking, not for cooking. It can be found in the tea section of most grocery stores or online.

While the collagen peptides are optional, they do help with the overall frothiness and texture of the Matcha. If you are vegan, you may omit the collagen.

This can easily be made iced. Be sure to use a liquid like MCT oil as your fat source. Ingredients like coconut butter will result in a clumpy beverage that's not very palatable.

PREP TIME:
5 minutes

COOK TIME:
10 minutes

YIELD:
2 servings

SWEETENER

- 2 cups (475 ml) full-fat canned coconut milk
- 1 cup (240 ml) chicken bone broth
- 3 tablespoons (15 g) cacao powder
- 2 ounces (58 g) dark chocolate chips or 100% dark chocolate, chopped
- 1½ tablespoons (22 ml) maple syrup (if using 100% dark chocolate)
- ½ teaspoon pure vanilla extract
- ½ teaspoon ground cinnamon
- ¼ teaspoon ground nutmeg
- ¼ teaspoon chili powder
- ¼ teaspoon kosher salt
- 1 tablespoon (15 ml) grass-fed butter or ghee (optional)
- 1 scoop collagen peptides (optional)
- 2 cinnamon sticks (optional)

bone broth hot chocolate

This recipe for hot chocolate will make you forget about any hot cocoa you've ever had. It's loaded with all kinds of nutrients like collagen, gelatin, protein, and healthy fats. Enjoy it first thing in the morning or whip some up as a nightcap. Or serve it to guests—I swear they will never taste the secret ingredient.

1 In a medium saucepan over medium heat, combine the coconut milk, bone broth, cacao, chocolate, maple syrup (if using), vanilla, ground cinnamon, nutmeg, chili powder, and salt.

2 Gently stir until the mixture reaches a low boil. Turn the heat to low and let it simmer for 2 additional minutes.

3 Transfer to a blender pitcher and add the butter and collagen, if using. Blend on high speed for 30 seconds and enjoy warm with a cinnamon stick in each mug, if desired.

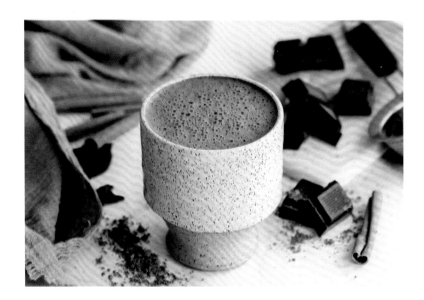

PREP TIME:
5 minutes

COOK TIME:
N/A

YIELD:
1 serving each

SWEETENER

mushroom latte, three ways

Mushroom lattes have been all the rage, and it's really no wonder why. They give you a steady energy flow without the crash, and they are herbaceous and delicious. Mushrooms have been linked to playing a role in boosting the immune system and improving liver function. Sounds like a win to me. If you're still not sure, try one of these three mushroom latte recipes—one hot, one iced, one either way—and you'll be hooked for sure!

CHAGA CARDAMOM

1 cup (240 ml) cold water
1 cup (240 ml) cold nondairy milk
2 tablespoons (32 g) creamy cashew butter
2 tablespoons (14 g) raw hemp seeds
2 scoops collagen peptides

2 teaspoons (10 ml) pure maple syrup
1 teaspoon (5 g) Chaga powder
½ teaspoon ground cardamom
½ teaspoon ground ginger

1 In the pitcher of a high-speed blender, combine the water, milk, cashew butter, hemp, collagen, syrup, Chaga, cardamom, and ginger. Blend on high speed for 1 minute, until smooth and creamy throughout. Taste for additional sweetener and pour over ice.

REISHI CACAO

1 cup (240 ml) boiling water
1 cup (240 ml) nondairy milk, warmed
1 tablespoon (15 ml) ghee, coconut oil, or MCT oil
1 tablespoon (15 ml) pure maple syrup or honey

1 tablespoon (5 g) cacao powder
1 teaspoon (5 g) Reishi powder
½ teaspoon Maca powder
Pinch of ground cinnamon
Pinch of pink Himalayan salt or sea salt

1 In the pitcher of a high-speed blender, combine the water, milk, ghee, syrup, cacao, Reishi, Maca, cinnamon, and salt. Blend on high speed for 1 minute, until smooth and creamy throughout. Taste for additional sweetener and serve hot.

MUSHROOM COFFEE LATTE

1 cup (240 ml) nondairy milk, warmed
⅓ cup (80 ml) freshly brewed coffee
2 teaspoons (3.6 g) cacao powder
1 teaspoon (5 ml) pure maple syrup

½ teaspoon pure vanilla extract
½ teaspoon Reishi powder
½ teaspoon Chaga powder
Pinch of ground cinnamon
Pinch of pink Himalayan salt

1 In the pitcher of a high-speed blender, combine the milk, coffee, cacao, syrup, vanilla, Reishi, Chaga, cinnamon, and salt. Blend on high speed for 1 minute, until smooth and creamy throughout. Taste for additional sweetener and enjoy hot or iced.

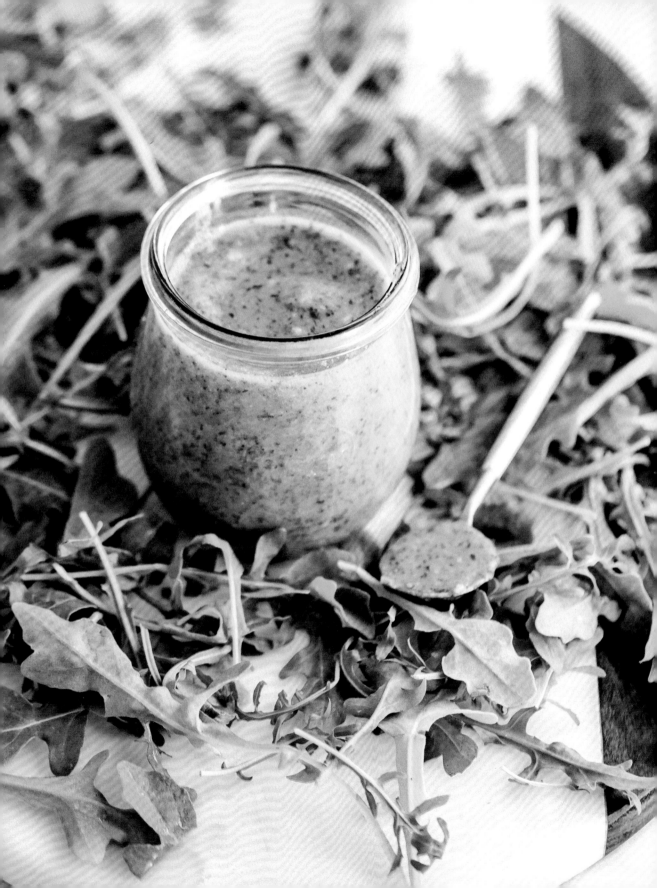

CHAPTER 9

sauces & dressings

LET'S CHAT ABOUT SAUCES AND DRESSINGS. These items often get overlooked, but in my opinion, they're some of the best things ever to make in the kitchen. They generally take very little time to prep and can enhance or even overhaul your meal.

You can create the base for a particular sauce, add an ingredient here, an ingredient there, and you have something else entirely. Doesn't that sound pretty spectacular? And what's better, when you make it yourself you know it's clean and wholesome, without any sneaky ingredients we don't want.

In this chapter, you will find classic sauces like an easy Clean Paleo Mayo, my go-to steak rub, and the best blender salsa of your life. You will also find more unique and intricate creations like Pumpkin Alfredo Sauce and a cashew-curry-cilantro sauce. Seriously, all these creations are going to knock your socks off.

◀ Arugula Pesto, page 183

cashew cheese

PREP TIME:
1½ hours

COOK TIME:
N/A

YIELD:
about 1½ cups
(350 ml)

1½ cups (225 g) raw cashews

1 cup (240 ml) filtered water

2½ tablespoons (9.3 g)
    nutritional yeast

2 tablespoons (30 ml) fresh
    lemon juice

3 cloves garlic, minced

½ to ¾ teaspoon salt, plus
    more to taste

½ teaspoon Dijon mustard

¼ teaspoon turmeric powder

Black pepper, to taste

This versatile cashew cheese can be used as a dip or sauce for pretty much anything—it's especially fabulous on my Cashew Cheese Chilaquiles (page 20).

1   Put the cashews in a bowl, pour boiling water over them to cover, and soak for 1½ hours. Drain and rinse the cashews a few times with cool water.

2   Transfer the cashews to the pitcher of a high-speed blender along with the water, nutritional yeast, lemon juice, garlic, salt, mustard, and turmeric. Blend until the mixture comes together as a thick sauce, scraping down the sides as necessary. You may need to add another tablespoon or two (15 to 30 ml) of water to help it blend together. The texture should be thick, but pourable. Taste for salt and add black pepper to taste. This can be stored in an airtight container in the refrigerator for up to 1 week.

slaw sauce

PREP TIME:
5 minutes

COOK TIME:
N/A

YIELD:
1¼ cups (300 ml)

SWEETENER

1 cup (240 ml) Clean Paleo
    Mayo (page 176)

¼ cup (60 ml) rice vinegar

2 tablespoons (30 ml) pure
    honey or coconut aminos,
    for Clean Paleo

¼ teaspoon kosher salt, plus
    more to taste

⅛ teaspoon black pepper,
    plus more to taste

This wonderful slaw sauce is delicious with a traditional cabbage coleslaw or mixed into my Brussels Sprouts Slaw recipe (page 130). Use it with your favorite salads if they need a real flavor booster!

1   In a small bowl, whisk together all the ingredients until thoroughly combined. Taste for salt and pepper. Store in an airtight container in the refrigerator for up to 5 days.

PREP TIME:
5 minutes
COOK TIME:
N/A
YIELD:
1 cup (240 ml)

SWEETENER

- ⅓ cup (80 ml) coconut aminos
- 3 tablespoons (45 ml) rice vinegar
- 1 scallion, chopped
- 2 tablespoons (30 ml) honey (see Note)
- 2 tablespoons (30 ml) sesame oil
- 1 tablespoon (8 g) sesame seeds
- 1 tablespoon (10 g) minced garlic
- 2 teaspoons (4 g) minced ginger
- 1 teaspoon (5 ml) fish sauce
- ½ teaspoon black pepper

NOTE:

To make this Clean Paleo compliant, omit the honey and add 2 extra tablespoons (30 ml) of coconut aminos.

asian marinade/ stir-fry sauce

This Asian marinade is so versatile; reduce it into a sauce or use it as a marinade for your favorite meats. Feel free to grill that meat, cook it in the pan, you call it. The flavors of ginger and garlic are really intense, in the best way possible, and you're going to love how much this marinade will heighten the flavors of your dishes.

1 In a blender, combine the coconut aminos, vinegar, scallion, honey (if using), oil, sesame seeds, garlic, ginger, fish sauce, and pepper. Blend for 30 seconds. Store in a sealed container in the refrigerator for up to 3 days.

PREP TIME:
3 minutes

COOK TIME:
N/A

YIELD:
about 1 cup
(240 ml)

clean paleo mayo

1 cup (240 ml) avocado oil
   or light-tasting olive oil
1 large egg, at room
   temperature
1 teaspoon (5 ml) filtered
   water
½ teaspoon Dijon mustard,
   at room temperature
½ teaspoon kosher salt
½ lemon, juiced, or
   1 tablespoon (15 ml)
   apple cider vinegar

The true magic about creating homemade mayo is that it is
the perfect base for many flavorful and incredible sauces
and dips. It tastes nothing like store-bought mayo, and I can
assure you that once you see how painless and easy it is to
make, you'll never look back. I highly recommend getting
your hands on an immersion blender, as this yields the best
results for me time and again!

1   Pour the oil into a glass jar (see Note). Add the egg, water, and
    mustard. Let settle for 1 minute.

2   Place an immersion blender into the container, resting it on the
    bottom, piercing the egg yolk completely.

3   Turn on the blender and leave it on the bottom of the jar for 20 to
    30 seconds, until the whole bottom has turned white.

4   *Very slowly* lift up the blender stick to continue emulsifying. This
    process should take anywhere from 30 seconds to 1 minute.
    Continue blending until the mixture has thickened to your liking.

5   Stir in the salt and gently fold in the lemon juice or vinegar. Store in
    an airtight container in the refrigerator for up to 7 days.

NOTE:

I use a 16-ounce (475 ml)
wide-mouth Mason
jar, and that has always
yielded the best results.
Use something that
just accommodates the
size of the stick blender
attachment.

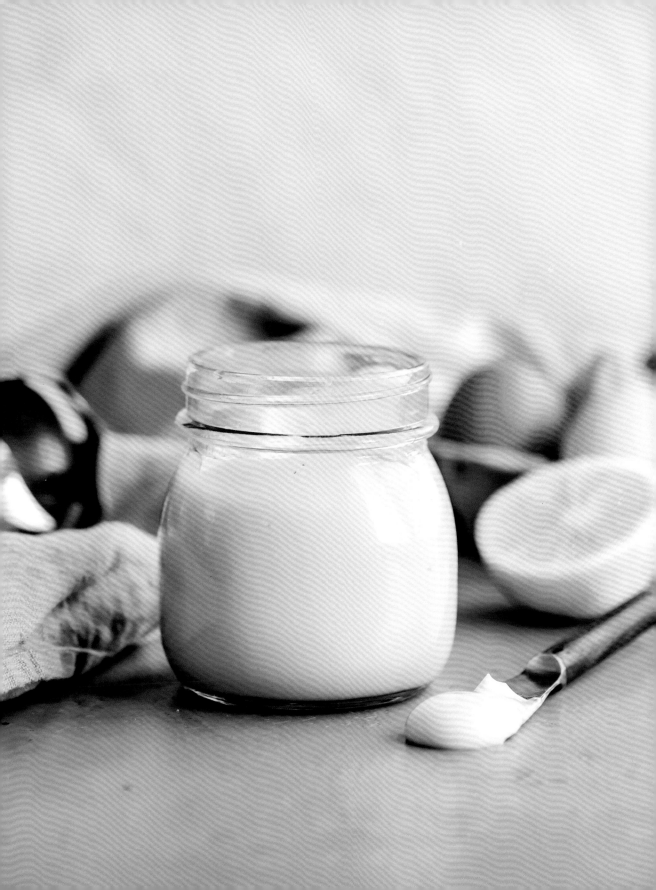

PREP TIME:
5 minutes
COOK TIME:
N/A
YIELD:
about ½ cup (120 ml)

SWEETENER

honey mustard sauce & dressing

HONEY MUSTARD SAUCE
½ cup (120 ml) Clean
   Paleo Mayo (page 176)
1 tablespoon (11 g) Dijon
   mustard
1½ teaspoons (6 g)
   whole-grain or spicy
   brown mustard
1 heaping tablespoon
   (15 ml) honey
½ teaspoon garlic powder
Black pepper, to taste
Sea salt, to taste

HONEY MUSTARD DRESSING
½ cup (120 ml) Clean
   Paleo Mayo (page 176)
1 teaspoon (4 g) Dijon
   mustard
1½ teaspoons (6 g) whole-
   grain or spicy brown
   mustard
1 heaping tablespoon
   (15 ml) honey
½ teaspoon garlic powder
1 tablespoon (15 ml)
   avocado oil
1 tablespoon (15 ml)
   filtered water
Black pepper, to taste
Sea salt, to taste

Let's kick everything up several notches by incorporating some of this fabulous two-for-one condiment in as many ways as possible throughout our day. It's so simple to whip up! Use it as a lovely dipping sauce for anything from chicken or roasted veggies to carrot sticks. Make the dressing for your favorite salad, and you will not be disappointed!

1 In a small bowl, stir together the mayo, mustards, honey, garlic powder, oil (if using), and water (if using). Taste and add salt and pepper to your preference. Store in an airtight container in the refrigerator for up to 1 week.

15-minute blender salsa

PREP TIME:
2 minutes

COOK TIME:
15 minutes

YIELD:
4 cups (950 ml)

6 Roma tomatoes, cut in half
½ white onion, cut into big chunks
1 handful cilantro
4 cloves garlic
2 jalapeños, cut in half (seeded for less heat)
¼ cup (60 ml) avocado oil
2 teaspoons (12 g) kosher salt, plus more to taste
1 teaspoon (1 g) dried oregano
½ teaspoon black pepper, plus more to taste

Who would have thought you could come out with such a flavor-forward and robust salsa without slicing, dicing, and roasting your ingredients?

1 In the pitcher of a high-speed blender, combine the tomatoes, onion, cilantro, garlic, and jalapeños. Blend on high speed until smooth.

2 In a medium saucepan over medium heat, warm the oil. Carefully pour the blender contents into the saucepan, while stirring. Add the salt, oregano, and black pepper.

3 Cook over medium heat, stirring frequently, for 15 minutes. It will become darker as the vegetables cook.

4 Taste for additional salt or pepper and transfer to an airtight container once it has cooled down. Store in the refrigerator for up to 10 days.

avocado aioli

PREP TIME:
5 minutes

COOK TIME:
N/A

YIELD:
1 cup (240 g)

6 cloves garlic
2 medium avocados, halved and pitted
½ cup (120 ml) Clean Paleo Mayo (page 176)
1 tablespoon (15 ml) fresh lemon juice
½ teaspoon kosher salt
⅛ teaspoon black pepper

This aioli is the perfect accompaniment to any meal. It's wonderful as a spread, but I also love to have it with my favorite cut-up raw veggies or as a delicious dip for chips or other snacks.

1 In the bowl of a food processor, pulse the garlic cloves multiple times until minced completely.

2 Add the rest of the ingredients and process on high speed until smooth and creamy throughout. Taste for additional salt and pepper. This can be stored in the refrigerator for up to 24 hours.

PREP TIME:
5 minutes

COOK TIME:
20 minutes

YIELD:
about 2 cups
(475 ml)

pumpkin alfredo sauce

¼ cup (60 g) ghee or
  grass-fed butter
½ yellow onion, diced
4 cloves garlic, minced
2 cups (475 ml) full-fat
  canned coconut milk
½ cup (112.5 g) canned
  pumpkin puree
1 teaspoon (2 g) white
  pepper, plus more
  to taste
1 teaspoon (6 g) kosher
  salt, plus more to taste
½ teaspoon garlic powder
2 teaspoons (5 g)
  arrowroot flour
1 tablespoon (15 ml)
  filtered water

Pumpkin alfredo sauce? I know what you're thinking. Why would I mix pumpkin into an alfredo sauce? Trust me on this one. This was my sister's recipe idea so many years ago, and I've been making it frequently ever since. I use it with eggs, roasted veggies, rice pasta—you name it. It is absolutely fabulous!

1 Warm a medium saucepan over medium heat. Add the ghee and let it melt completely. Add the onion and cook until it appears translucent, 4 to 5 minutes. Add the garlic and cook for 1 minute, until fragrant.

2 Add the coconut milk and whisk until well combined.

3 Mix in the pumpkin, pepper, salt, and garlic powder. Whisk over medium heat until it reaches a low boil. Lower the heat to a simmer and cook for another 10 minutes. Remove from the heat.

4 Transfer the alfredo to a blender (or use an immersion blender). Blend on high speed for 30 seconds, until smooth. Return to the saucepan.

5 Make an arrowroot slurry by combining the arrowroot flour and water in a small bowl. Add to the alfredo, whisking well. Add salt and pepper, to taste.

6 Store in an airtight container in the refrigerator for up to 1 week.

PREP TIME:
5 minutes

COOK TIME:
35 minutes

YIELD:
about 1½ cups
(350 ml)

bone broth gravy

4 cups (950 ml) bone broth
2 large yellow onions,
    coarsely chopped
8 to 10 cloves garlic
4 sprigs rosemary
2 tablespoons (30 ml)
    coconut aminos
Kosher salt, to taste
Black pepper, to taste
2 tablespoons (30 ml)
    grass-fed butter or ghee
2 tablespoons (30 ml)
    organic heavy cream or
    coconut cream
2 tablespoons (16 g)
    arrowroot flour
2 tablespoons (30 ml)
    filtered water

I'll be the first to tell you that the holidays are not the only time you need the perfect gravy recipe in your life. This bone broth gravy is incredibly nutrient dense, flavorful, and should absolutely be enjoyed year-round (as frequently as possible!). I like to pour it over anything and everything, as I don't need to worry about it containing anything that would make me feel less than fabulous!

1   In a medium saucepan, combine the broth, onions, garlic, and rosemary. Bring to a boil over high heat, then lower the heat to a low simmer. Cover with a lid and simmer until the onions and garlic are soft, 30 minutes.

2   Add the coconut aminos and add salt and pepper to taste.

3   Transfer the ingredients to the pitcher of a blender. Add the butter and cream. Blend on high speed until well combined, 30 seconds.

4   In a small bowl, create an arrowroot slurry by whisking together the arrowroot flour with the water until smooth.

5   Transfer the gravy to a large bowl. Very slowly whisk in a little bit of the arrowroot slurry at a time, until it reaches your desired thickness. Serve warm. Store in an airtight container in the refrigerator for up to 3 days.

NOTE:

To reheat the gravy, pour it into a small saucepan over low heat and whisk until warm throughout.

PREP TIME:
5 minutes
COOK TIME:
N/A
YIELD:
about 1 cup
(240 ml)

tomato-garlic aioli

1 batch Clean Paleo Mayo
    (page 176)
¼ cup (65 g) tomato paste
3 cloves garlic, sliced

My husband asks me to make this aioli as a dipping sauce for everything from roasted veggies to scrambled eggs. Oh, and it's the perfect pairing for my Patatas Bravas (page 76).

1 In a wide-mouth Mason jar, combine the mayo with the tomato paste and garlic. Blend using an immersion blender until smooth and creamy throughout. This will take 15 to 20 seconds.

2 Taste for seasoning and store in the refrigerator in an airtight container for up to 1 week.

PREP TIME:
5 minutes
COOK TIME:
N/A
YIELD:
about 1 cup (240 ml)

triple-c sauce

⅔ cup (100 g) roasted
    cashews
½ cup plus 1 tablespoon
    (135 ml) full-fat canned
    coconut milk
½ cup (25 g) packed cilantro
1½ tablespoons (22 g)
    coconut aminos
2 limes, 1 zested , 2 juiced
2 heaping teaspoons (30 g)
    red curry paste

This cashew-curry-cilantro sauce is a real dream come true. The roasted cashews really play well with the fresh flavors from the cilantro and lime. In addition to Easy Beef Lettuce Wraps (page 119), use it as a dip with cut-up raw veggies or pour it over the Cauliflower Rice Meatballs (page 124).

1 In the bowl of a food processor or high-speed blender, combine all the ingredients. Blend until completely smooth and creamy, scraping down the sides as necessary, adding more coconut milk if needed to thin.

2 Store in the refrigerator for up to 1 week.

PREP TIME:
5 minutes
COOK TIME:
N/A
YIELD:
about 2 cups (475 ml)

DAIRY

arugula pesto

2 cups (40 g) tightly packed arugula
1 cup (90 g) finely grated Parmesan cheese
½ cup (75 g) pine nuts
1 tablespoon (6 g) lemon zest
2 cloves garlic
1 teaspoon (6 g) kosher salt, plus more to taste
1 cup (240 ml) extra virgin olive oil
Black pepper, to taste

This pesto is going to become your new favorite condiment. I am notorious for mixing it with my Clean Paleo Mayo (page 176) for the most delicious pesto aioli ever. I love adding this pesto to salad dressings, eating it with roasted veggies, and more. It's very quick and easy to make, and I cannot wait for it to become a staple in your kitchen.

1 In the bowl of a food processor, combine the arugula, Parmesan, pine nuts, lemon zest, garlic, and salt. Process for a few minutes until finely chopped.

2 Very slowly drizzle in the olive oil while processing on high speed. Taste for extra salt and add pepper to taste.

3 The pesto will keep in the refrigerator for up to 3 days, but be sure to cover the top with a very thin layer of olive oil to keep it from turning brown. It will also keep in the freezer for up to 3 months.

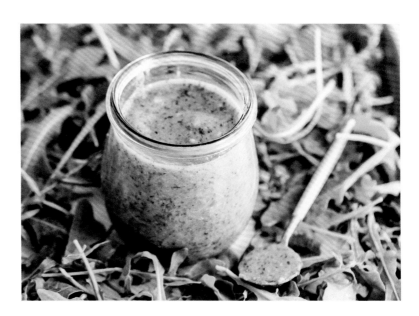

PREP TIME:
5 minutes

COOK TIME:
35 minutes

YIELD:
4 cups (950 ml)

tomato cream sauce

¼ cup (60 ml) extra virgin olive oil

1 small yellow onion, diced

4 cloves garlic, minced

2 cans (28 ounces [794 g]) whole peeled tomatoes, coarsely chopped, juice reserved

6 sprigs fresh thyme

1 tablespoon (18 g) kosher salt, plus more to taste

2 teaspoons (1.4 g) dried basil

2 teaspoons (6 g) garlic powder

2 teaspoons (4.8 g) onion powder

Ground black pepper, to taste

2 cups (475 ml) full-fat canned coconut cream

¼ cup (60 g) grass-fed butter or ghee

2 teaspoons (5 g) arrowroot flour

2 teaspoons (10 ml) filtered water

NOTE:

I found the best flavor develops when I set aside about 1 cup (240 ml) of the red sauce before continuing with the recipe. It's still delicious on its own and can be used like any marinara sauce.

If you're looking for a super flavorful but simple-to-make tomato cream sauce, this is your ticket. Though it's made with canned tomatoes, you would never ever guess. It's simply luscious. You're going to want to pour it over everything, but I recommend tossing it with your favorite pasta or zucchini noodles or slathering it over grilled chicken or shrimp. It's straightforward, creamy, and so full of flavor that nobody will have any idea there isn't any real cream in it.

1 Heat the oil in a large saucepan over medium-high heat. Add the onion and cook, stirring well, until lightly browned, 7 to 8 minutes.

2 Add the garlic and cook for another minute, until fragrant.

3 Add the tomatoes with about half of their juices (discard the rest). Add the thyme, salt, basil, garlic powder, and onion powder.

4 Bring the mixture to a boil. Reduce the heat and simmer, uncovered, until the mixture has thickened, 15 to 20 minutes.

5 Remove and discard the thyme sprigs. Taste and add more salt and black pepper if needed. Transfer 1 cup (240 ml) of the sauce to a container and set aside to cool (see Note). The plain tomato sauce can be used in other recipes.

6 Add the coconut cream and butter to the mixture in the saucepan.

7 Create an arrowroot slurry by whisking together the arrowroot flour and the water in a small bowl until smooth. Slowly pour the slurry into the sauce while stirring continuously until thickened, 1 to 2 minutes. Remove from the heat.

8 Store it covered in the refrigerator for up to 3 or 4 days. It can be frozen for several months as well.

PREP TIME:
1 minute

COOK TIME:
N/A

YIELD:
¼ cup (30 g)

best steak rub

4 teaspoons (24 g) kosher salt

4 teaspoons (8 g) black pepper

2 teaspoons (5 g) smoked paprika

1 teaspoon (3 g) garlic powder

1 teaspoon (2.4 g) onion powder

There is nothing better than getting the perfect flavor on your favorite cut of steak, am I right? I'm a rib-eye kind of gal, and when I use this dry rub on it and cook it in a cast-iron pan with lots of fat, I feel like I am unstoppable. (Hungry for it? See page 118.) This seasoning is not only perfect for steaks—I love to use it in my eggs, on sautéed veggies, or on other proteins, too. It's so versatile and absolutely phenomenal!

1 In a small glass jar, add the salt, pepper, paprika, garlic powder, and onion powder. Stir well or cap it and give it a good shake. Store in a dark and cool cabinet for up to 6 months. Use liberally!

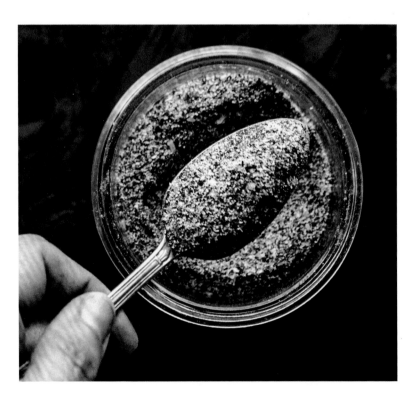

acknowledgments

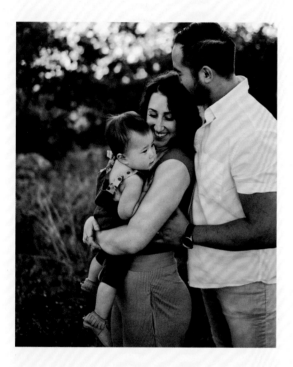

TO YOU, THE READERS: I would not have written this cookbook if it weren't for the constant encouragement, support, and kind words I receive from my readers and followers. Thank you for reading my blog, trying my recipes, and always leaving me with honest and constructive feedback. Thanks to you, I have grown so much as a blogger, photographer, author, and person. You push me each and every single day, and for that, I cannot say thank you enough.

TO SOPHIE: My firecracker, spunky, sassy, incredibly bright baby girl. I still look at you sometimes in complete awe, wondering how it's possible that you are real. I learn so many new things from you every moment of each day we spend together. You have taught me specifically to hold more space for myself and how to be more patient, wild, and free (simultaneously somehow!). Every dance party, every snort sound, each giggle, wanting "mo" (more) of everything you eat . . . it all fills up my cup with so much joy and bliss, it's insane. This first one and a half years of parenting has not been an easy feat, but you make every trying day and emotionally vulnerable experience beyond worth it. I can't wait to continue bonding with you over our shared love for food. This is all for you, sweet girl. You're my moon and stars.

TO TIM: From holding me while I cried after dropping tons of food on the floor to being my never-ending garbage disposal, to being the person that changed my "I can'ts" to "you will's"—thank you for that. Nobody in the world can be as gracious and accepting of my failed recipes as you can. You still polish them off, so there is zero food waste, but you willingly let me know, "You've really missed the mark here. Yuck." You have always been my biggest supporter. Everybody knows that I'm the one with my head in the clouds, dreaming of all the things I want to accomplish and provide for us. You are the grounded one that is full of so much logic, patience, and insight it *still* blows me away every dang day. You have never ever cast any doubts on me; having someone right next to me throughout this process, who believed in me every step of the way, has made this incredibly beautiful, enjoyable, and rewarding. Thank you for never ever, even for one glimmer of a moment, not believing in me. I couldn't accomplish all that I have in my life and in turn, with this cookbook, without such an incredibly insightful, compassionate, loving, and strong man by my side.

TO MY MOM: As far back as I can remember, you have been such a cheerleader for me, and you truly champion me every day of my life. In your mind, there were never any limitations to what I could accomplish. Growing up and far into my adulthood, you were always the first person I'd come to with my greatest moments of joy as well as in the most painful phases in my life. The amount of gratitude I want to give you is completely immeasurable. Transitioning out of the corporate world and setting forth on my own journey to success has been so much easier knowing you'd hold my hand every step of the way. Thank you for the countless numbers of hugs and kisses. Thank you for calling me almost every day just to say "hi" and make sure I'm doing well (especially during the book-writing process). Most of all, thank you for being the best example possible for what a mother and successful and strong woman should look like.

TO MY SISTER: Through thick and thin, you have proven to be the most inspiring little sister ever. I know that usually it is the little sister who is supposed to look up to the big sister. However, I find myself looking up to you every single day. I have always turned to you for advice, as your opinion means more to me than you know. Thank you for styling me from head to toe during my photoshoots. Thank you for giving me a thumbs up or thumbs down for my clever or not-so-clever recipe ideas. To spending hours upon hours on Pinterest with me, driving to my house in the middle of the night to help me, and wiping away my tears of frustration when a recipe didn't turn out the way it was supposed to—I could never ask for a more supportive, selfless, creative, or gracious little sister. So many of the recipes in this cookbook were created thanks to your unwavering support and insight, and for that, I am forever thankful.

TO QUARTO: In particular, Jill Alexander, Meredith Quinn, Heather Godin, and Todd Conly. Wow, has your team ever received so many questions? Thank you for keeping up with my persistent and endless inquiries. Your replies always left me feeling at ease and more comfortable with my journey ahead. Moreover, thank you for taking a chance on me. You all have contributed so many ideas to help make my book even better than I could imagine. Thank you for all of your excitement, most of all. Having a team as supportive, understanding, and patient as you all has made this into an incredibly joyful experience.

about the author

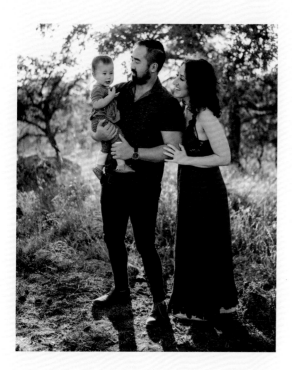

MONICA STEVENS LE originally began cooking with the vision to help those closest to her achieve their lifestyle goals. She wanted to show people that the only way to live their lives to the fullest was to feel like their optimal selves, every single day. Her recipes and cooking styles are mainly influenced by her grandmother's Mediterranean and Jewish recipes, in addition to Asian flavors thanks to her partner's side of the family. For the most part, though, Monica enjoys playing in the kitchen and creating her own flavor profiles.

She is the founder of *The Movement Menu*, a whole-food blog that exhibits many paleo-friendly recipes that won't break the bank. She does not believe that we need to eat perfectly in order to reach optimal health and wellness. Perfection is not sustainable long term, and she wants her readers to change their lifestyles instead of going on a strict or "perfect" diet. Monica originally started her blog as a way to share her ideas with close friends and family. It wasn't until she was laid off from her sales position in the corporate world that she decided to pursue blogging, cooking, and writing full time.

Aside from spending a lot of time in the kitchen, Monica enjoys traveling, spending time with her family and friends, and being outdoors. Her primary goal has always been to inspire others, leading them on a path to changing their lifestyle and improving their day-by-day quality of life.

index